Companions for the Passage

MARJORIE RYERSON

Companions for the Passage

Stories of the Intimate Privilege

of Accompanying the Dying

University of Michigan Press :: ANN ARBOR

Copyright © by the University of Michigan 2005
All rights reserved
Published in the United States of America by
The University of Michigan Press
Manufactured in the United States of America
⊚ Printed on acid-free paper

2008   2007   2006   2005   4   3   2   1

A CIP catalog record for this book is available from the British Library.

Library of Congress Cataloging-in-Publication Data

Ryerson, Marjorie.
    Companions for the passage : stories of the intimate privilege of
accompanying the dying / Marjorie Ryerson.
        p.   cm.
    ISBN 0-472-03078-7 (pbk. : alk. paper)
        1. Death—Psychological aspects—Case studies.   I. Title.
BF789.D4R94   2005
155.9'37'0922—dc22   2004024018

To my children, Emily and Nicholas

With gratitude for their unwavering friendship and love

Acknowledgments

I would like to thank the many people who have shared their stories of accompaniment with me as well as the others who have supported and encouraged me forward in the journey of assembling this book.

I am indebted not only to those whose stories appear on the pages of this book but also to the many other people whose stories—for space reasons alone—could not be included in this volume. They include: Peter Voelker, Jessica Mazariello, J. Donald Schumacher, Tessa Cone, Dr. Denise Niemira, Jerry Thomas, John Morton, Virginia B. Newman, Priscilla Baker, Henry Isaacs, Ila Washburn, Nancy Dubois, Roberta Dean, Diana Peirce, the Rev. Timothy Eberhardt, Prudence Berry, Mark Lewis, Deborah Straw, Melvin H. Mandigo, Connie Cadow, Penny Brooks, Margot, Douglas Wilson, Anne Lorda, SallyAnn Silfies, David Shepler, Dr. John Delaney, Larry Roberts, Sarah Howell Skarrow, Kendall Farrell, Andrew (Dito) Staley, and Tracy Chipman Kavaney.

I also wish to thank the key people who have guided and encouraged me as I assembled *Companions for the Passage*. They are Dr. Joseph O'Donnell, Dr. Patricia Boston, Dr. Clare Wilmot, Penelope Graham, R.N., Dr. Robert Johnson, Dr. Howard Jonas, Dr. Martha Regan-Smith, Marie Kirn, Donna Sultura, Gina Sonne, and Virginia Fry.

Contents

xi   Foreword by Thomas Moore

1   Introduction

9   Marlene Petrucci

20   Donald Hall

38   Julie Morton

54   Tim Palmer

72   Letha E. Mills, M.D.

89   Anita F. Bonna

101   Amy Silverberg

108   Ann Schauffler

123   Archer Mayor

129   Margaret Robinson

139   Frances M. VanDaGriff

153   Diane D. Guerino

166   Ira Byock, M.D.

Foreword
By Thomas Moore

Ever since I published *Care of the Soul* almost twelve years ago, people have been asking me, "What is the soul?" Each time, I'm silent for a moment. There is no adequate answer. I mumble a few words that I hope are not too abstract, but I realize immediately that they are far too inadequate. What I could do in response would be to give the inquirer a copy of this book by Marjorie Ryerson. If you want to know what the soul is, be a witness to the death of a loved one or even someone you don't know.

The lively, emotional, and thoughtful stories in this book reveal to the reader the very essence of what it means to be a visitor on this planet. The sense of connection, purpose, wonder, and mystery intensifies at the moment of death so that the witness can't help but be educated, in the deepest sense of the word. You discover that human life at its core is something you can never understand fully and can't control. You learn the importance of being present to another. You sense that somehow nature is in accord with the most intimate events in your life. You may have an intuition that the dreams that have drifted into consciousness night after night during your life may have been significant after all.

As a witness, you may be affected for life by the passing of someone you love. Throughout this book you'll find the words *sacred* and *spiritual* used sparingly to sum up the atmosphere of a peaceful death. Each death has its own shape and rhythm. Each is its own ritual. In the presence of death you stand at the edge of eternity and discover something of the essence of your own life.

My mother died last summer. She had had a minor stroke and then a hemorrhage in her brain. The last real conversation I had with her was a telephone call between these two events. She was nine months dying. From the time I left home at thirteen to enter a seminary, I have always lived at a distance from my family. During her last illness, I visited my mother many times and spoke to her in her dementia and massaged her and sat silently with her for hours. When the end came, my wife and I had been teaching in England and were making a brief visit to Ireland to be with friends and relatives. As my mother died, I lay in bed in that country of her origin, talking to her inwardly across the ocean.

My father and I had discussed many times whether I should stay within reach. He thought I should go on living my life and spreading my message, one that he understands and supports. When I still feel some guilt about not being present at my mother's death, I remember my father. He is a deeply emotional man, but all his life he has taken an unsentimental position on everything, especially in matters of life and death. When my mother's condition first worsened, the staff at the nursing center called a meeting with the family. My father arrived with an agenda all typed up and copied. He passed it around to the surprised nurses, dietician, and chaplain and called the meeting to order. He asked for specific information and told them warmly but firmly that he wanted no heroics in keeping my mother alive. In his mind, she had begun her departure long ago.

We Americans live in a society where the people are full of heart but where the way of life is lacking in deep romance, mystery, ritual, and heartfelt connections. I think we treat each other badly—especially groups that are in any way different—because of our materialistic and mechanical view of life. We don't see through to the person beneath an accent or skin shade. Medical students are trained in a purely physical view of the body and are not always educated in the mysteries of illness, dying, and love. To be present at the death of our loved ones, we sometimes have to fight the system and deal strenuously with emotionally cool technicians and arrogant medical personnel. We have to be warriors defending the needs of the soul.

But sometimes a grace intervenes. When my mother was at the very end, the family called for a priest. No one could ever be as devout a Catholic as my mother, who was born on the feast day of the Annunciation and was named Mary Virginia, Virgin Mary. She said a rosary every day of her life, and when I was sorting through her things later, I found several well-worn devotional cards with prayers for a happy death. In the hospital room, the elderly priest arrived, whipped out his harmonica, and played the tune "Going Home," by Dvořák. My father, a musician and equally devout Christian, said he couldn't have imagined a more beautiful death.

I wish everyone would read the stories in this book, feel them, take them in, and be affected by them. We all need this kind of education in soul. If we knew death with this kind of intimacy, maybe we would pause before advocating wars, even on behalf of freedom and peace. Maybe we would be radical initiators of conflict resolution at home and abroad. Maybe we would honor the precious lives of children who need to be educated in the human sensitivities described here. Maybe we would get over our religious excesses and prejudices and discover how deep a spiritual way of life really is. Maybe we would learn that nature is more intimate to us than we ever like to think and needs our care and protection.

The people who tell their stories in this book are incredibly alive to human connection. Their memories of love and loss have in them lessons that perhaps can only be learned by witnessing death. I believe that if we could all be exposed to these lessons, the world would be a far better place. For we learn from death how to live, and we prepare for our dying by the way we live.

Introduction

I was blessed through much of my adulthood to live near my parents. That proximity, however, meant that as my elderly father endured the last difficult months of his life, I was the person he telephoned each day whenever he needed anything. My father's requirements grew increasingly complex as his health failed. I spent as many hours a day with him as I could, keeping him company, helping out, playing music for him.

My father and I had embarked on this intimate, final journey two years before, when his once-athletic body began to fail him. Even though he had robustly survived many decades into old age, I found myself living in fear of losing him. Medical tests gave us diagnoses of multiple myeloma, congestive heart failure, prostate cancer, and early emphysema. He fell regularly, often suffering serious injury. When I arrived at his house each day, I never knew what new crisis I might find. I never knew if his tenacious will to live would prevail or if the multiple diseases in his frail body might take him by evening.

My father resented having to rely on anyone else, including his children. Even more acutely, he detested the string of indignities being forced upon his body. But as debilitating pain from cancer raged in his bones, he fought a bitter, losing battle against disease and old age. I asked various health-care professionals what I should expect as his condition deteriorated further. How would I recognize when death was imminent? What should I do for him when that time arrived? Medical personnel had few answers for me. One doctor said my questions were impossible to answer. Another doctor admitted that the sight of death so terrified him that he had always tried to avoid it. My father's primary-care physician told me that even after seeing patients through life and death for twenty years, he was unable to predict death with any exactitude. "Besides," the doctor said with obvious affection and hope, "he's a tough old bird. Perhaps he'll pull through this and live to see one hundred." But with a long list of incurable diseases, it was clear that my father had no prospect of returning to full health.

My mother had died many years before. Although I had helped out during her illness, I had not been by her side at the moment she died. And throughout her long illness, someone else—my father— had been in charge. But this time around, the front line of defense was sick. This time, I was the one who needed to know how to recognize when the time was near and exactly what to do when it arrived.

My father fielded health crisis after health crisis. He was in the hospital. He was home. He was back in. During his hospital stays, I would discuss pain medications with the attending medical staff. We would fret over doses and counter-indications. We would keep track of how much he did or didn't eat. We would discuss his inability to negotiate walking, and other signs of his physical deterioration. We would tally the number of hours he had slept the night before. We did not discuss death.

In late May, my father left the hospital to attend my daughter's college graduation. We dressed him in his gray suit and borrowed a wheelchair. He was back in the hospital by day's end, exhausted but happy. That trip was his last into the outside world.

During the next six weeks, he grew visibly weaker by the day. His eyes did not see well enough to read. He hated television. So he lay in bed, waiting for me to arrive. Day after day, he and I floated through the same slow, exquisitely tender rhythm. He often expressed a desire to leave the hospital, but he was dependent on a complex network of medical interventions, well beyond what I could provide for him in his house or my own.

Early one July morning, a nurse from the hospital telephoned me to say that my father was having trouble breathing. I was in nightclothes, baking bread in my sunny kitchen. I was on vacation from my teaching job and feeling especially grateful for the stillness and freshness of that summer morning. "Trouble breathing," I thought?

"He's had asthma for years." But I knew the nurse wouldn't have called me if the situation hadn't been critical.

I got to the hospital as quickly as I could and spent the next several hours sitting quietly with my father as he struggled for breath. His doctor arrived at 10 A.M. on rounds, drew me out into the hall and gently said to me, "Your father may make it through today, but he may not. It would be a good idea to call your brother and sister. I think this is the day you've been asking about. This may be the day we lose him."

After calling my family, I returned to my father's side. We talked very little during the next few hours, but his eyes said a great deal, communicating a mix of anxiousness and concentration. My father seemed distracted by the work required to breathe. He stared upward, toward the ceiling. He sometimes would rest his hand lightly against mine but then pull away as soon as my fingers responded. He could not seem to stay connected. I didn't know what he was thinking, but I felt enormous respect for his ability to focus on what he felt he needed to do. Most of the time, the two of us were completely alone. A warm breeze was billowing the curtains of the room's French doors, which were open to the Hospice garden just outside.

Shortly after 1:00 P.M., my father looked directly at me, his eyes clear. He spoke for the first time in hours. "I want to go home," he said. I paused, wondering what he really meant. But I chose to respond literally. "You can't go home right now, Daddy," I told him. "You're too sick. You need to stay here just now. But I'll stay with you. I won't leave you."

Those were his last words. After that, he was turning inward, toward a place I could not follow. My brother quietly slipped into the room at 1:30, gave me a hug, and then pulled a chair up to the other side of the bed. He and I sat in nearly silent vigil, resting our hands on our father's arms. My sister lived five hundred miles away; she was on her way, but it would be hours more before she arrived.

Just before three in the afternoon, my father's breathing became very shallow, as if the air was going no deeper than his throat. "I love you, Dad," my brother said urgently. "I love you, Daddy," I echoed.

My father drew in three rough breaths, each separated by a long pause. Then his head jerked slightly to the side and settled back on the pillow. He lay still, his mouth open. We waited. We waited. He did not breathe. I'm not sure whether my brother or I breathed in those long seconds either. But we were there together. Our father was not alone.

Although the hospital room suddenly filled with activity—a nurse feeling for a pulse, a minister saying a prayer—my instincts told me to not break contact with my father's body. I sat motionless, my hands against his still form, wanting only to comfort him wherever he was in those moments just beyond breath. I gently rested one hand on his arm and the other on his shin, overcome with love for him. I was so connected to him at that moment that I felt as if I had walked over the edge of life with him, right by his side. As I sat there, I was startled to have the sensation that my father's life energy was pouring into my hands and filling my body. The unknowable was happening, and I was participating to the fullest extent that I could.

Within minutes after he stopped breathing, the sky filled with massive storm clouds and the blue sky vanished. The wind picked up speed. Lightning broke the darkness. I finally allowed myself to lift my hands from my father's body, but my sense of connection to him did not change. I rose and moved, but I felt as if I was carrying my father with me. It was distressing to separate from his still form.

That evening, when I called my son in Boston with the news, he said that at 3:00 that afternoon, outside his office building, the peaceful summer afternoon had dramatically shifted. Lightning and winds had moved in and the sun had disappeared. He said that he had paused at work, watching the sky, and wondered if his grandfather had just died.

In the weeks that followed, the anguish of the loss of my father was buffered by an almost tangible sense of existence having become surreal. I functioned in a fog, trying to comprehend small details that I had previously taken for granted. In those hard weeks, however, friends and acquaintances reached out to offer embraces and remembrances. I was initially surprised by how many of them asked if I had been present at the moment of my father's death. At first I thought they were merely curious, but I soon discovered that all the people who asked that question of me had also witnessed the death of someone they loved. They wanted to support me. But they also wanted to share their own stories with someone whom they thought could understand what they, too, had been through.

By listening to their stories, I gained a sense of clarity about my own experiences at the time of my father's death. I learned from their stories, as I had learned at my father's bedside, that the witnessing of the transition from life to death is the most powerful experience we can have. For many of us, it is also a profound privilege. After hearing those initial stories from friends who had accompanied loved ones at the time of death, I felt inspired to reach out to others to collect the stories for this book. I gathered many more stories from generous people than could fit into this one volume, and each of the stories was unique and significant.

Almost all of us have heard stories like these; by a certain point in our lives, all of us have told them. The telling and retelling of these stories from the final days and hours together is far more than a ritual. The stories about the end of life that we share become a significant part of our efforts to make the loss manageable. No one who has been through such an event ever forgets it. Even decades later, the smallest details remain. We remember exactly who was present and what each person said and did. We know, by heart, the dying person's smallest gestures and last words. The processing and sharing of these experiences enables us to better understand death, to accept the changes it brings, and to cope with the inevitable grief.

Such stories may teach us about death, but they also teach us about the very finest love and connection possible in human relationships. These stories are examples not only of challenging sacrifice but also of the deepest rewards possible. These stories teach us how to be open to this remarkable journey. They teach us about what truly matters.

—Marjorie Ryerson

Companions for the Passage

Marlene Petrucci

Marlene Petrucci, an R.N., was with her mother Mary, also an R.N., through the months of her mother's illness from cancer as well as at the time of her death. A hospital social worker originally introduced me to Marlene, telling me that Marlene's story was remarkable. Indeed, I found Marlene herself remarkable, too. Her training as a nurse had prepared her for her mother's illness, but it was Marlene's openness of heart that allowed her to embrace the experience of losing the person she loved most in the world.

My mother, Mary, was sixty-seven when she was diagnosed with cancer. She knew that she had cancer long before it was diagnosed. She was an oncology nurse at our local hospital. She started the oncology program there, which is ironic. Being a nurse, she knew her own body; she knew something was very wrong. I had noticed some mental changes in her, and being a nurse myself, I thought, "Oh, maybe she's having little strokes, little TIAs." But being her daughter, I said, "This can't be happening to my mother."

We went to many different doctors together. The doctors said, "The lump on your skull is just old-age bone growth, Mary." "The pain in your joints is just arthritis." "You're just getting old." She wasn't buying it. She took me down the street to Pleasant View Cemetery. She showed me where she wanted to be buried. She said, "I have cancer, and I'm going to die."

I was thinking, Mom! You look healthy. You look good. You're walking every day. You look good. What are you talking about? But she was finally diagnosed. By that time, the cancer had metastasized from her lungs—she had it in both lungs, throughout all of her lung fields—to almost every bone in her body. It was even in her sinuses. The cancer was everywhere but below her knees and below her elbows. Doctors even suspected the cancer had spread to her brain as well. They said she could expect to live about four months.

Being the person that she was, she said, "I have always told my patients to go ahead and do chemotherapy because it can decrease the pain." And she was in a lot of pain. So she decided to do chemotherapy, and it did help with her pain, it did help extend her life. She lived a total of nine months from the time she was diagnosed. But it was hard; my mom was my best friend. We used to do so much together. She would come to my house for dinner several times a week. We'd go shopping. We'd go out for meals. We did a lot together. And for those nine months, my sister and I took care of her.

Actually, it was a great nine months in many respects. I say to some of my patients whose family members have contracted cancer, "You know, the time can really be a gift to you. It's kind of like finding a pearl within an oyster, what you can get out of it."

In those months, my mom and I had tremendous talks. We shared a lot of feelings, very honest, intimate feelings. My mother would say to me, "I'm really going to miss spring. I'll miss the mountains and the sky and the sunshine." I was able to say to her, "I'm proud of what you have done. I'm proud of you as a mom for what you have accomplished." All those little things are important to say.

When you stop to look at it, we all go through day-to-day chores and work and lives, and we rarely stop to say to the people in our lives just what they mean to us. We don't notice all the little things that we should appreciate. When you're with somebody who's ill and you don't know how much time she has, it can bring meaningful, very real rewards. If you use that time well, you can live—in those months—years!

Of course my mother did not want to die. She fought it all the way and was in denial for much of that time. She wasn't going to die. She was going to beat this thing, even though being a nurse, she knew otherwise. So she wouldn't listen to the doctors when they would say, "The X-rays look worse. The cancer has spread. We need to try this. We need to do that." So I carried a burden that way, if you can call it a burden. It was a time of a lot of joy and a lot of living as well as a lot of suffering. One of her oncologists said to me, "Probably you are suffering more than she is with this, just trying to deal with her pain, her emotions, her knowing that she's going to die." Yes, it was hard, but it wasn't difficult in the sense that I begrudged her. In fact, taking care of my mom was wonderful in her last few weeks, especially the last week.

Death is something we all go through. We all have to exit the same door. My mother finally came to terms with the fact that this was it. Her own body was failing. She was having a very difficult time breathing. Her anxiety over not being able to breathe was just terrible. We couldn't get her undressed. Here was this woman who was just so into how she looked. Goodness, if there was a spot on her shirt, she would have to change it. And we couldn't get her out of her own clothes.

When my mom took a severe turn for the worse, she'd been on oxygen for quite a while. Her physical needs had increased to the point that we couldn't take care of her at home, so we brought her in to the hospital.

In her final three weeks in the hospital, we would sit and watch the birds come to the feeder outside the window. Mom believed that people who had died watched over us, that their spirits were really never dead. Mom had been good friends with Phil, the hospital's CEO. They had worked together. She had helped take care of Phil when he was dying from cancer. She recounted to me a conversation with Phil in which he said that he loved birds, especially cardinals. He told her how infrequently he could get red cardinals to come visit. So my mother felt that birds at her feeder were from Phil. To her, the birds were something spiritual. One day a red cardinal came to the feeder, and she said, "Oh look, isn't that beautiful? That's from Phil."

Her close friends came in to the hospital to visit her, and she began saying her good-byes. That was probably one of the hardest things to see and to hear. She finally said—and I think this is very hard for most people who are facing death—"I am ready."

The last five days were very much a blur in some ways. We started her on a morphine drip, trying to make her comfortable. We would give her whatever she wanted. She was pretty conscious up until the last couple of days. She never, unfortunately, got to a point where she was comfortable.

In those final days, my mother would talk out loud from the place that she was in, wherever that place was. I don't know where people go when they get to that place between consciousness and unconsciousness. I've pondered that a lot. I don't know whether people go back in time to when they were children. I don't know whether they go to a place that we are just not aware of, somewhere between earth and whatever else is out there after life. There's just this time period in which I know that hearing is the last sense to go, or so they say, medically. My mother could hear the outside world, but she herself was in a different place. She oftentimes would not respond to questions. But I sat with her. I was there twenty-four hours a day, and we talked, or I talked with her and lay on her bed, beside her, and thought about how the tables had turned. I found that was a very interesting thought—in just the feelings that it brought—that, in death, we all change. She brought me into this world. She gave me life. She took care of me and raised me, and here I was, helping her to die, doing all the things that she used to do for me when I was a child. And that was hard. It was hard because I wanted her to hold me, to simply be a mother for one last time. And yet, through all that, those needs of mine had to be placed aside.

Instead, I would be the one holding her hand or rubbing her back or rubbing her shoulder or putting a cold facecloth on her. I would be the one trying to give her little sips of water to moisten her mouth. It was very hard to realize that this person whom you have known ever since your existence started on the face of this earth was, in a short period of time, never going to be here. I could not fathom that. I could not comprehend life—the world—without the presence of this woman in it.

My grandmother, my mom's mother, had been dead for fourteen years. My mother would call out to her, asking her for water or saying, "Mom. Mom. I can't wake up. Help me wake up." Articulately. Very clearly. She was talking to her mother, as if her mother were present. It was extremely painful to hear. I think it was painful for her, too, because I felt that maybe she wasn't ready to die. Maybe her saying to her mother, "Mom, I can't wake up," was actually her not wanting to pass on.

My mother's goal throughout her illness was always to make it to a holiday, to make it to a birthday or something like that. Her final goal was to live until Easter. She had been born on Easter and she wanted to make it until Easter. I would say to her, "Mom, it's Wednesday. Easter's four days away." And she would yell out, "Easter, Easter." It was very interesting to hear sometimes what she would fixate on and what she would hear and respond to.

I think many people choose the time of their passing, but not all people. My mother could have held on longer. She could have died earlier. When she finally passed, it was beautiful in the sense that my sister was there, my husband was there, and a lot of her friends from the hospital with whom she had worked were there, too. We were all sitting on her bed or standing beside her bed and we were telling stories of my mother working at the hospital. We were sharing the funny stories of things that had happened, such as the day they were trying to put a Foley catheter in a patient and this went wrong and that went wrong. We were telling the stories and everybody was laughing and *that's* when she passed away. It wasn't a time when people were crying. It wasn't a time when it was silent. That was the time she chose. It just fit in with her personality. She always loved to laugh and loved to tell funny stories and jokes. That was the atmosphere in which she really loved to be. That's the way she wanted it to happen, whether it was for her or for us. And she had made it. She had made it to Easter.

Her burial had to be postponed, due to our great New England springs where you can't get up to the cemetery because it's all muddy and covered in snow. So instead, we buried my mother in May. It was May 10, the day before Mother's Day. It was kind of a rainy day, and we buried her half a mile from my house, in Pleasant View Cemetery. The day that we buried her, it got very cold in the evening. My husband and I decided to drive up to the cemetery to put a cover over the flowers at her grave. We got out of the front door of the house, and there was this bird. You're not going to believe this story. There was this bird. We'd never heard it before.

We'd never seen it. And to this day, we've never seen this bird since.

The bird's cry sounded like something between an owl and a loon, a very distinct call. And we remarked, "I wonder what kind of bird that is. I've never heard it." We went up to the cemetery, a half mile away, and the same bird was at the cemetery. It had followed us. The cemetery gate was locked at the bottom so we had to walk up. We covered all the flowers to protect them from frost and walked down again. The bird stayed above us, calling. I said, "Let's get into the van. Lock the doors as quick as we can." It really shook me. We got back down to the house, and the bird was at the house. It had followed us home.

The bird stayed for about three weeks, maybe a month. It only appeared in the very late evening, in the dusk of the evening, when it was too dark for us to see it. The bird was always flying around in the air above us. Sometimes it would be down the road, but we would hear it from the house. It would be flying around, but we never could see it. We never saw this bird! The bird stayed around for maybe three weeks, maybe a month. And then after that, it left. It disappeared. I felt that it was a kind of symbol; my mother was released from the world of her suffering. By burying her, she was finally free of this world.

Mother's Day this year, May 10, was exactly the same day and the same month we buried her, one year ago. On this Mother's Day, my husband and I had been outside all day long. That evening, we drove to a city, forty miles from here, to pick up my husband's teenage son. We got back home about 8:30–8:45 in the evening. We stepped out of the van, and the bird was back, crying above us in the darkness. My husband grabbed me. He said, "The BIRD!" And I said, "The BIRD!" I got goose bumps. I could feel the hair rising on my arms.

Just like the year before, we couldn't see the bird. We never saw it. It was flying around and it was calling. And then it left. It was only there that night, and we haven't heard it since. People can say what they want. My husband, who does not believe in anything like that, was even struck by the experience of it. The first night we heard it, the night of the burial, the bird's presence was frightening. But when it came back on Mother's Day this year, it made me cry.

I know it's corny, but I can't help but feel that in some way, somehow, that bird is a gesture from her. I think her whole death brought me the sense that there's something much greater out there than what we feel or even than we think is out there. I believe that the whole human spirit is so much stronger than we know. I just cannot put it into words.

I have been with several people when they died, the moment that they've died, and I've been with people who have died since my mom's passing. And you know, you *know* the moment that they die, especially with my mom. I knew the exact second that she passed. Medically, I can say, "Oh yeah, there are color changes. There are temperature changes. There are little things like that." But there's something deeper than that. There's something—the soul, the spirit. It's gone. You can just tell. I think one of the biggest things in death is that you can really feel the absence. And it's not an absence of life. It's an absence of—I don't know what. I've never been able to find the words for it. There is a housing that is left, a shell, the house that kept the soul, that kept the spirit, and you can just feel that the spirit is gone. It not just that the *life* is gone.

There is certainly a part of me that is so different now that I can only say is influenced by my mother, by her death. Maybe it is that I've taken on a part of her. I don't know. Her death has been the saddest thing that I have ever experienced. The grief, at times, is almost unbearable, but going through her death with her has given me so much insight and understanding. It has profoundly changed my life and how I think. I'm now trying to enjoy life, trying to do everything that I can, so that I will never look back and say, "Oh, my God, I wasted my life. I'm facing what my mother faced, and all I did was work." So I changed to part time at work; I work two twelve-hour shifts a week. That's a huge change. I feel what I give my patients is so much deeper than where I was and what I could give before.

For my patients who have their spouse, their mother, their father diagnosed with cancer, or even when the patients themselves are, I've shared my experiences with them. They have asked me questions, and I've shared with them some of the details of my mother's illness and what went on between my mother and me. There's something that's deeper in me now. It's not nursing, it's caring. It's sharing, and on a much, much deeper level. After something like this, you're in tune with a whole different part of yourself, of life, and of everything.

Through her illness, through everything, it seemed that my mom's whole life changed. Here was somebody who had been unhappily married for years and who had suffered emotionally with that, even after her divorce. And finally, she became like a flower— you plant it and you simply watch it grow. She was like a child again. It was like she had been reborn. She just blossomed.

She started the cancer center, and she just loved it; she loved her patients. She started doing all sorts of things that she loved and found interesting. She became a whole new person in the span of eight or ten years. It was so sad to see that life that she had, that was so perfect for her, be shortened by this illness.

She would ask, "Why? Why me?" She was a very strong, devoted Catholic and certainly believed in God, though she doubted her religion toward the end. She had led her life by the Bible. She was human; she had made mistakes, but she had led a good life. She had helped others. And she wondered why God was taking it away from her when she had finally found a life that she loved so much. She wanted so very much to live. How could anything take that away from her?

She said, "Why? Why now? Why couldn't they have found this earlier?" That was a question that she kept asking me. She asked "Why now?" so frequently that it was often on my mind. I worked at the large medical center about an hour away. I would be driving home, and in that hour of commuting time, I'd be thinking. One day, the answer kind of came to me out of the blue, and the next time my mother asked, I shared my thoughts with her.

I'm not religious; spiritual, yes; religious, no. But I said, "Mom, number one, maybe, though, God *was* looking out for you. Think of all the things you have done in the last six years. Think of the fun you had in Las Vegas. Think of going with Joe to California and flying over the Grand Canyon. Think of learning how to play golf and how much you love that and have loved that, and how you have gone out every day and played. Think of the oncology clinic over the last three years. Look at all you have done. If they had diagnosed this two years ago, three years ago, you wouldn't have done all that. You would have missed out on so much because you would have been going through chemotherapy or radiation therapy. Maybe someone *was* watching out for you. I can understand the question, 'Why me?' Why is this given to you? I don't know. But maybe the fact that it wasn't diagnosed four years ago, three years ago, two years ago was indeed a gift because you would not have done the oncology program. Look at all the people whom you have helped. Look at all the people whom you've touched—their lives, their families."

I think my saying that made a difference to her. I think hearing that and having her understand—Yeah, you're right. I would have missed out on that—made a difference. How much of a difference, I don't know.

We had a lot of those close conversations. But those are the blessings along the way. Oh, it's incredibly sad, of course. I still cry. But I don't think I would have changed it. As much as I miss my mother, I am thankful for that time, because we shared some great things. I was bringing her into the hospital one day, and she said, "You know, Marlene. I'm really proud of you as a nurse. You're a much better nurse than I ever could have been." That type of thing—would we have shared that? I don't know. I don't think so. The time was really limited for us. We would go out. I would take her for walks when she would want to, or we'd just go out and do things. She was in a wheelchair. All those little things that you can do are just such gifts because they are so appreciated. It felt so good to be able to do those things for her.

I felt a lot of suffering for my mother. Just seeing this woman who had been so independent and had done everything for herself and who had walked every day, to then be wheelchair-bound, her body swollen, and with no hair. Yet she found dignity and quality in that life. I suffered more with her losses of independence, I think, than she did.

It was just so painful to see a person who was so sick and who had so much cancer in her body just want to keep doing everything she could possibly do, and living each moment, and trying so hard to live, so hard to beat the cancer. When she died, that kind of suffering over her condition stopped; the grief encompasses relief. I think that's something that's very hard for people to understand and to accept, that that relief is actually okay to feel and that it's very normal. The relief comes in so many ways. It's not only getting your life back. Your suffering stops and begins in a whole new way. It was just draining. It was so draining. I was relieved, too, that her suffering was over.

Grief is intense and complex. When my husband's father died, I came back from where he lived and went back to work. My supervisor came up to me and said, "How are you doing?" And I said, "I don't know how I'm going to do this. I have lost three people in a year that are very dear to me. I don't know where it's going to come from. How am I going to get through this?"

It just looks so big. You're not just grieving for that person. I wasn't just grieving for my father-in-law; I was grieving for my mother. I was grieving for the passing of her brother. All of these losses just gathered and gathered and gathered. It became just so huge. Today, I have made it beyond that point. I don't know how I ever did it. All I can say is that I think human beings are remarkable. The inner strength that people can pull up is amazing. But grief really stays with you in some forms. It pops its head up in very, very strange ways. It makes you sit and do nothing. It makes you clean the whole house. It drives you. Yet sometimes you say, "Why do I feel the way I do? Why do I feel such low self-esteem?"

I was actually talking to a friend yesterday. I said, "My self-esteem has just been shot. I don't know what's wrong." And she had lost her mother, too. And she said, "You know, Marlene, it's grief. It's the loss of your mother." And I said, "You're right. That's the person who was always there for me. She was the person who could hold me, love me, give me that."

My mom wanted us to take a vacation once she passed away. And we did, last year. My husband and I took two weeks and went to Hawaii. It was wonderful. We probably wouldn't have done that otherwise. It was extraordinarily expensive, but you know, we're going back again in two months! Being part of a death makes you so aware of life, of what you want to do, and how you want to live. I love my job. I love what I do. I wouldn't change it. But it's not my *life*. It's not what I want to do every day. That was one of the big things I learned.

I've talked with my patients and they say, "Well, we were planning this trip—" One person wanting to go to Alaska said, "Now I won't be able to do it." And I said, "Why won't you be able to do it?" "Well, because I was diagnosed with cancer." And I said, "Just because you were diagnosed with cancer doesn't mean you can't take the trip. You need to take the trip. Your family needs to take the trip. It will be one of the most incredible experiences of your lifetime. It will be something for them to look back on and have, forever."

What an experience, being part of a death. What a trip. I don't know if there was anything spiritual or not. I look back and think of all the things that we laughed about, of all the things we did, of my mom, through her illness, always having a sense of style. Her makeup had to be just so, even though she was so bloated. She had no hair, no eyebrows, no eyelashes. But I would do hats for her, and pins. I'd do her makeup for her, and it was just so much fun. It was almost like both of us were being children. We had a lot of good times together.

There was an oyster, and it had a pearl, and the pearl is all those memories.

Donald Hall

As a poet, I had long followed the writing careers of both Donald Hall and his wife, Jane Kenyon. One year, a close friend of mine, knowing that I was assembling material for my own book on death, gave me *Without,* a book of poems Donald had written in response to Jane's death from leukemia. After reading the book, I decided to track Donald down and ask him if I might interview him. He graciously agreed to meet with me in New York, where he was teaching poetry for a semester at New York University. When we met, Donald gave me a copy of his wife's posthumously published book of poems, *Otherwise.* In the title poem in the collection, Jane describes her day-to-day activities while living with Donald: walking the dog, writing poetry, sharing meals—all with the knowledge that some day, "it will be otherwise."

Jane and I were married in Ann Arbor, where I was a professor. We had our busy-nesses, lots of people around, and students and so on. After three years we moved to New Hampshire, and I went free-lance. Now there were just the two of us alone in the same house all day, both writing poems. I was also writing other things, to make a living, but not so much Jane. We had what I continually call a double solitude. We were extremely close—we were doing the same things in the same house. In order to do that, we had to make a lot of boundaries. But we didn't quarrel. Maybe once every four years we had a quarrel. But we were kind to each other.

I would meet her in the morning when we were both writing. We'd both come for a cup of coffee at the same time. We wouldn't even speak. I would just pat her on the ass. We were enormously comfortable together, so comfortable that we didn't need to talk about it. We never talked about our relationship. Jane suffered from depression, and often I was able to be helpful. When she was in the pits, it was a trouble, but it was not a trouble between us.

I was nineteen years older than Jane. In the past, we had decided not to get married several times because we thought she would be a widow for twenty-five years. In those years, I worked very hard writing children's books. I did four books a year, some years. I intended to leave her an estate so that she could stay at the farm and live after my death. She might well have supported herself by that time, but I wanted to make sure. I wanted to be the *mensch*.

When she was thirty-seven, she had a cancer of the thyroid gland. It was totally encapsulated. It was taken out. Nothing ever happened. That's the first time we faced the possibility of her death. Then a few years after that, I had colon cancer. I had just turned sixty-one. So we then faced my death, which we had expected all along would come first. My chances of survival were fairly good. My chances were 60 to 70 percent of living five years. But then, two and a half years later, the cancer metastasized to my liver, and I lost two-thirds of my liver, and my chances of living were down to 30 percent. Some people think less. But it's been about seven years since then. I was considered cured two years ago.

In 1993, Jane climbed Mt. Washington. We went to India for a month. We were constantly doing poetry readings together by this point because she was beginning to get well known. We traveled a lot, doing readings. It was the most active year of our lives. Probably the best year of the twenty years at the farm was the year we will remember least, because everything was routine. We adored routine. We would get up at 5:00, and I would bring her a cup of coffee. I would start working at 6:00 and she'd start working at 6:30, and we'd have an early lunch. All summer, she would garden in the afternoons while I went back to the desk. Our lifestyle was uninterrupted. There are no cocktail parties or dinner parties in rural New Hampshire.

Jane and I were very close. We lived alone and were very satisfied in each other's company. We were sort of reclusive. She was originally more reclusive than I was. I followed her, as with so many things, into a greater reclusiveness. We invented people we called Elmer and Mary who were the excuse we gave as to why we couldn't go out on a Saturday night. If invited somewhere, we might say, "Oh, too bad. Elmer and Mary are coming," or "Sorry. We're going over to Elmer and Mary's house."

We went to church on Sundays, but for the rest of the week, we mostly just saw each other. The neighbors and cousins were very good at not coming or calling. They were afraid we were writing, and we let them think so—and besides, we *were* writing a lot. That year was so active. Then in January 1994, we went together to Bennington, Vermont, to read our poems and to lecture. It was the last time we read together. Jane was happy there, and we did well. When we came home, she began to get flu symptoms. I was doing a reading with Geoffrey Hill, who was a dear friend of hers as well as mine, but Jane wasn't able to come. She had bone pain. She just felt rotten. A lot of people who have leukemia begin by thinking it's the flu.

I went away to Charleston, South Carolina, to read by myself on January 29. I kept calling her up and saying, "How's the flu?" First, it was worse and then it was better. I flew back on January 31 and arrived late because of plane equipment trouble. I called Jane from the airport and said, "How's it going?" And she said, "Oh, God, I had a terrible nosebleed, a humongous nosebleed. I went to the hospital and they stopped it, and now I'm waiting for blood work. And then I went out and the car wouldn't start!" Later on, when she was writing in a little notebook, she wrote, "I thought my trouble was that the car wouldn't start."

This is so strange, but when I was in the phone booth, talking to her, the sentence flashed into my head: Jane has leukemia. I had never known anyone with leukemia, but I might, sometime, have read that bone pain, nosebleeds, and hemorrhages can be associated with leukemia because cancer cells knock out the platelets.

I swung by to see my mother, who was in an old-folks' home attached to New London Hospital, where Jane had been for her blood work. I walked in to see my mother. A nurse came in and said, "Dr. Foote wants to see you." I knew what he was going to tell me, and he did. So I went back to my mother and said, "I've got to see Jane. She has leukemia." And my mother—her brain worked fine, but she kept thinking I had said "anemia," not leukemia. Anemia is something she had had when she was a child, and she recovered from it. That's probably why she kept turning the word into anemia.

By then, Jane had had transfusions. A neighbor had driven her. She was in terrible shape. Initially, our attitude was, Well, what have we got ourselves into? Oh boy. Shortly after, I learned that the raw results for grownups with leukemia were 50 percent survival, 50 percent death. Then we learned that her particular case was much worse. She had the child's kind, from which 95 percent of children now recover. It's called ALL—acute lymphoblastic leukemia. But when you get it when you're forty-six years old, your chances are not as good.

And then we learned that a particular characteristic of the DNA called the Philadelphia chromosome was in her cancer cells. Its presence means that chemotherapy can never save your life. Only one thing can possibly save your life, a bone-marrow transplant. The bone-marrow transplant has a kind of rejection effect on the cancer cells, but only 15 percent of the time. So her chances were poor.

One of the terrors of her leukemia, for both of us, was that my cancer would come back and I wouldn't be able to take care of her. There was a very good test for the presence of a metastasized colon cancer, a blood test, and I could take that every now and then. But when I was ready to take the test, we were both frightened because the second-most important thing, after the disease itself, was the relationship between the two of us, the caregiving relationship, independent of the goddamn leukemia.

Jane exemplified a role model for me in lots of ways. She had taken care of me when we thought I was going to die. My illness was not protracted. After my liver came out, I was walking around in a few weeks. I got better quickly, but we were just waiting for the cancer to come back and for me to die. It was different after Jane got sick. She was terribly sick for fifteen months. And in those fifteen months, there were only two or three weeks when she could actually revise a poem.

There was no bone-marrow match in Jane's family. At moments, she seemed about to die. Jane's mother died while Jane was sick, as did my mother. Jane had pneumonia in March, just after my mother died. The pneumonia was PCP, which AIDS people get all the time. Finally, we found an anonymous bone-marrow donor near Seattle. In September, we were set to fly out to Seattle for the transplant when the leukemia came back. Jane was put into remission in about three weeks by chemo, but we knew the remission would not last.

Finally, we were able to make the trip to Seattle. After the bone-marrow transplant, when she was so damn sick, vomiting eight, ten times a day, in terrible pain, she would say to me—she called me Perkins—she would say, "Perkins, am I going to live?" And the rest of the question was, "Are we going through this shit for nothing?" By the way, it was always "we." It was "we" with liver cancer. It was "we" with leukemia. It was absolutely ours and we weren't self-conscious about saying that. I would always answer, "Living is what we're here for. That's what we're trying for." I didn't say, "Yes, of course you're going to live." I couldn't stand that. Neither of us could stand cheerfulness. We always hoped that she would live, but neither of us said, "Of course I'm going to live," or "Of course you're going to live." There was no bullshit.

When she was in Seattle, I was in a nearby apartment. I would go home and wash her sweats—she'd go through three in a day because there would be blood and vomit on them—and then I'd get ready to go back the next day. Of course I would do everything for her that I could. When she was back at the apartment, I learned how to do infusions through her Hickman, the heart catheter. I'm a technophobe, and for me to learn how to program a pump was something. I was just terrified: I was sure that I couldn't do it. But of course I could.

After a bone-marrow transplant, all you can do then is cross your fingers. The new marrow tries to reject the body it's in. Many people die of BOD, which is beno-occlusive disease. BOD shuts off the liver as the new marrow rejects the liver. That didn't happen. So she was getting better. We were told it would take about two years for her to be normal after the transplant. That's the usual time. For some people the time is quicker. But she had skin problems and neuropathies. Most of her pain was from the treatment after the leukemia.

Her pain levels were at nine or nine and a half out of ten. When she had previously been so sick at Dartmouth-Hitchcock Hospital and in great pain, she had ranked her pain at four or five. At hospitals all over, they ask, "On a scale of one-to-ten, what is your pain?" This time, she was at a nine and a half.

The depression that she had suffered from and written about so eloquently disappeared. She wanted to live. She was so surprised how much she wanted to live. She often had written wonderful poems about depression when she was coming out of it. She did have one incident of depression in Seattle that was probably partly caused by the drugs. For most of the fifteen and a half months of her illness, however, she was not depressed in the clinical sense. Of course she was unhappy. This situation she was going through was phenomenal.

I used to read Henry James aloud to Jane all the time, but not when she was sick. After she got ill, one Dave Barry column was a good day. Her mind didn't work very well. When Jane was totally out of it, when she was asleep, I would write. When she would see me writing, she would say, "Perkins, what are you doing?" She was glad somebody was writing. So I read aloud to her some of my poems about her and about her illness, including one called "Without," which was originally *not* about her death but about the landscape of the illness itself, that terrible landscape. She liked it. She liked hearing about it.

When I had been so sick, after the liver cancer, she had brought me the manuscript of her poem called "Pharaoh." It is a marvelous poem. It is about her waking up at night and seeing me lying still on my back with my feet poking up like a sarcophagus: "And beside him, the things he would need in the next life, his glasses, his book." She showed it to me, and she said, "Perkins, do you mind?" I said, "Well, it's a little weird, but I love it. It's a beautiful poem."

So then I had the same experience that she had had. She had written about looking ahead to my death. We knew I might die. And then I was writing about the landscape of her illness and the daily events. I wasn't writing out of expectation that she would die, even though both of us knew that her chances of survival were poor. Many of her late poems have to do with my impending death and her impending widowhood. The end of the title poem of her book *Otherwise* says "One day it will be otherwise." And it *was* otherwise.

The illness drew us even closer than we had been. At one point during Jane's illness, a social worker said something to me like, "Why don't you go away for a few days, take a holiday." I just was dumbfounded at that notion. I wanted to spend every minute with Jane that I could. We didn't do anything self-consciously, but I overheard people saying to each other, "Do you see the way they look at each other?" Apparently our devotion to each other was kind of legendary. But there was nothing else to do. You're certainly not choosing an alternative.

It seemed to me that we became one soul in two bodies. And again, we didn't chatter much. God knows she couldn't. But we could look at each other. There were times that I couldn't touch her because she required such isolation. That was very hard. She had no immune system whatsoever. And I certainly couldn't touch her much because she was in so much pain. Jane was out of her head sometimes, but not very often. I did all that caretaking, and I loved it. She kept saying, "Perkins, I can't get over you. I can't get over you." I was not putting gold stars on my forehead, I promise you. I was just utterly, utterly, twenty-four hours a day, into this caregiving, caretaking, helping.

After getting home from Seattle, we kept having to go up to the hospital to get her blood checked. At first, three times a week. Then twice a week. Then once a week. On April 4, her blood looked good. On April 11, we went up and the blood was drawn. No longer from her Hickman—she didn't have it any more—but from her arm. They had pulled out the Hickman because she couldn't have any more chemo.

The blood was drawn from her arm, and we went upstairs to the infusion room to wait. It took a long time to get the results, but it sometimes did take a long time. We weren't particularly suspicious. But for several days, she had been feeling worse and was having more bone pain. The day before we had bought a new car, and she had insisted on coming with me to sign for it. She was in terrible shape that day. The leukemia was back, but we didn't know it. She'd been in terrible shape from time to time, all along. It wasn't a smooth recovery. When we bought the car, she took five minutes to sign her name. Her hands were disabled by one of the anti-rejection drugs called Cyclosporine. We took the new car and drove to the hospital.

We were waiting and waiting. I commandeered a bed for her because she felt so bad. We were supposed to sit down and wait.

Jane went to sleep. A nurse came in and took her vital signs. Then another nurse came in and told me to go see Jane's doctor. I did, and found the oncologist sitting down. She looked at me and said, "The leukemia's back. There's nothing to do." She burst into tears. So did everybody.

Jane probably cried less than anybody else over the news. They gave us a pack of tissues to take back in the car. Jane had walked into the hospital; it was hard for her to walk in, but she was trying to build up her strength. But there was no point in strength-building any more; we took the wheelchair out. We drove back home, knowing that she would die. We both were weeping in the car, in the brand-new car.

When we got home, I took Jane inside and then just took the phone off the hook. I didn't want one of the children to call at that point. I would call them later. We lay in bed together and hugged and wept and thought about what we had to do. We had, as it turned out, eleven days. I had asked the hematologist, "How long?" I had asked all sorts of questions, "How long and why now?" Jane had asked only one question, which was, "Can I die at home?" And her doctor said, "I don't see why not."

Jane's oncologist came to the house twice during the eleven days that Jane took to die. The doctor didn't need to do that; she obviously couldn't do anything. But we knew what we had to do. Jane said a couple of things to me that afternoon. She said, "I don't fear punishment by God." What she *didn't* say, and I couldn't say, was, "I'll see you in heaven." We didn't know about heaven. I was skeptical, more than she was. She may have been skeptical at that point, but she wouldn't even discuss it. But she talked about where she wanted her archives to go. And then we knew we had to finish her book. It hadn't been started. Her publisher had already said the next book should be a *New and Selected*. Her way back to poetry was going to be to fashion this book as the new and selected poems. I had Xeroxed all the pages from the old books, for ease in sorting through and cutting out and so on. This was something we had to do, and we had to write her obituary and plan the funeral service.

She was determined to do it all right away, and she was absolutely correct because she lost the power of speech after four or five days, or virtually lost it. At the end, you couldn't tell how much she was aware of. So we went to work and created the book.

I'd say to her, "Maybe you could leave this poem out," and she'd say, "Yes." Then I'd say, "This one ought to be in," and she'd say, "I don't think so." I'd read it aloud to her. Sometimes she'd say yes and sometimes no. I did not argue. She sent me upstairs to where all the new poems were. There were more than we had both remembered. There was one I'd never seen. It was a wonderful poem. And she said, "Oh, I thought that little thing was never going to be anything." We talked about the book's sequencing, and we made the decisions. We worked maybe two or three hours that second day. We even worked the night of the first day. I put the phone back on the hook and told my children and told her brother. When she went to sleep, I called people—her best friends and so on—to tell them. The next day we worked about three hours on the book until she got totally exhausted. The day after that, she was feeling horrible. I said, "Let's wait." And she said, "No, we have to do it now." And we did it.

We also wrote her obituary, each contributing to it and revising it. I got the hymnbook and we chose hymns. I said that I wanted two poems, "Otherwise" and "Let Evening Come," to be read. I knew somebody could do it. I couldn't do it. Well, maybe I could have, but I didn't want to do it. I'm a planner, a relentless planner. We sort of planned for everything. Actually, we never talked about the gravestone, which was strange. But I kept planning. It's a form of fending off the reality, to plan for the reality.

Jane and our dog, Gussie, were totally devoted to each other. I said, "When Gussie dies, I'll scatter his ashes on your grave." She said, "Oh, that will be good for the daffodils. Perkins, what will you think of next?" And she laughed. We laughed two or three times. But she also wailed twice. Just twice. She said, "Dying is easy. But the separation—" One of those times she said, "No more fucking. No more fucking." And then she screamed. Otherwise, she was much quieter than I was. She was very deliberate.

In one of her poems about her father, Jane described how dying people put their hands out on the bed, but she writes that you must not try to hold them, you must let them go. Well, I still touched Jane sometimes and slept next to her while she was dying. The two things that she loved most in the world, besides poetry and me, were flowers and music. She couldn't have flowers when she was sick because they bring bacteria in. I played music for Jane all the time. And it was black women's voices or Messiaen. I played music by a lot of people whose names begin with *M,* like Mendelssohn. In those last days, I wanted to play music, but Jane wouldn't let me. She said, "No."

Thirty-five or forty bouquets or plants arrived. She wouldn't have a flower in the room. She was letting go. It was painful for me. It is painful. She didn't want, except for me, the things that held her to life. That would make her want to live too much, and she didn't want to feel that. She wanted to let go. She wanted to die sooner rather than later, once she knew she had to die. They could have put her in the hospital, by the way, and kept her alive an extra month, in terrific pain. Nobody wanted to do that. Nobody suggested it. We didn't want it. We knew she was going to die. So we did all those practical things.

Maybe the third and fourth day, of the eleven days, she said, "There's something I need to tell you. I want. I want. I want spinach. No, that's wasn't the word." And I kept thinking, Eat? Drink?—because of her word spinach. And then she stopped speaking on purpose because she couldn't stand to have something that came out be stupid or to not be able to say what she wanted to say. So I then asked her questions that could be answered yes or no. Or I would say, "I love you, and I know you love me. You don't have to say it." I kept saying this mindlessly, over and over again. But she did say it, too, when she could. And it was just a caress of course, saying "I love you" was just a caress. It wasn't giving information or news or anything.

Even when Jane was no longer in command of language, she could still manage to communicate some. Liam Rector is a poet and a dear friend, and his wife, Tree Swenson, was Jane's designer for her last four books. Jane did five books, but Tree began with number two and went on to the posthumous one.

Liam and Tree drove up to say good-bye. They lived extremely close to us, in Somerville, Massachusetts. But Tree knew there would be this posthumous "new and selected" volume called *Otherwise,* and she said to Jane, "Do you have any ideas about the cover?" Tree always worked from a painting or something for the cover. And Jane said, "Yes," but she couldn't speak to tell the name of the artist. And she said, "It's in the living room." I put Jane into the wheelchair and wheeled her into the living room, and that was the last time I did that.

I can't remember what day it was, but it was halfway through those eleven days. I wheeled Jane out to the living room and she pointed at the book. She knew it was there. And it was a book that someone had sent us at Christmas, in Seattle. It was a book about the Impressionists' gardens, and I remembered then, sitting in that apartment in Seattle, that Jane had said, "That would make a nice cover."

Since she couldn't use her hands, I just flipped through the book until she pointed. In that way, she contributed to her book design. Tree took the book, and I never asked for it back. I would like Tree to keep it. And it is a very beautiful cover, the cover of Jane's book. That was just one thing, a relatively good thing that happened during the eleven days of her dying.

Wednesday night to Thursday morning was the worst time because she still could mumble but she was out of her mind. That's when I was lifting her on to the potty. Oh, she'd wet herself every now and then, and then try to get up and go. And I would lift her onto the potty with her arms around my neck. I'd put her arms around my neck, and she'd say "Mama, Mama, Mama" to me. I'd leave the room and when I would come back she would be across the room. She couldn't walk, but she got across the room. I was terrified that she would break something and add to her pain. I was still thinking that she might live another month. I called up the hematologist at 6 A.M. and said, "Get her a bed. We've got to get her in." And the hematologist said, "Okay, you get the ambulance. I'll get the bed." And I came back to Jane and I said, "I've got a room. You've got to go back to the hospital." And she wept. She said, "Do we have to?" I said to Jane, "No, we don't," and I called the hematologist back.

I'm a bossy type. I kept interfering medically. Jane wouldn't remember all she'd been going through in the last few hours. I could always make a list and tell them everything. But then I would sort of suggest connections, as if I were a medical researcher or something. I heard myself doing this one time, at least. I know I was a presumptuous bore to all of them.

After we got to using diapers, Jane never got out of bed again. The second or third day of those eleven days, I took her out of the house one more time, for her to sign a new will. But that was the only time she left the house after we came back from the hospital. She didn't leave the bedroom after that or even get out of bed. She used diapers.

Over fifteen months, I'd become a great scholar of her face and of the pain that she was suffering. We did get some morphine, when she couldn't move any more, and taped the needle to her leg. She couldn't roll over. Every now and then, she'd moan and I'd give her a shot. But I really don't think that she was in that much pain.

My sense of her departure was one of dissolution. Cell by cell. I'd seen her go through so much acute suffering. And there had been high moments of anxiety for various reasons during the illness—when she turned blue and so on—when I thought, She's dying. But now she really was.

It happened slowly, over eleven days. It happened just absolutely progressively. There were no ups and downs. She just went down. Hair by hair, cell by cell, she was disappearing. And I knew she would. After all, we had both been practicing for this for quite a while, as we had with me, too, but much more with her because it was fifteen months of bad odds. Now we knew it was happening. I didn't want to hurry it up; she did want to hurry it up, and I understood that. I didn't resent that. But I continued to feel protective and caring, although I knew I was losing her.

The day before she died, her friends came to see her and say good-bye. My children came to see her to say good-bye. I would leave them alone together. One of the things with Jane was that she had to sort of lift herself up, which was painful, to be able to think and speak. The day before she died, her dearest friend, Alice Mattison, who is a short story writer and novelist, helped lift her up when a nurse's helper was scrubbing down her back. Alice said to Jane, "This isn't much fun, is it?" And Jane said, "No."

The morning of the last day, I had been gone, getting a newspaper or something, while the nurse's aide was with Jane. And when I was gone, Jane thought that I was dead. So I was careful thereafter. I didn't leave her except to take a piss or to grab something to eat, and I'd eat it in front of her, of course. I said to her, the noon before she died, when somebody was with her, "I'm going out to put the mail out." And she said, "Okay." Her last word.

That night, the Cheyne-Stokes breathing started. I knew about it. My grandmother had had Cheyne-Stokes when she was dying. Every now and then, I'd kiss Jane, in spite of the injunction in her poem against touching the dying. I'd just peck her. About 8:00, I kissed her lightly, and she kissed me back. I don't think kissing is autonomic.

That afternoon, on Friday, the day before she died, fifteen bunches of flowers arrived. Also Bill Moyers sent, Express Mail, the dummy of the book about poets and poetry, with a full-page picture of Jane. Alice Quinn, poetry editor of *The New Yorker,* faxed us. She was accepting five poems by Jane. So I said to Jane, "You have five poems coming out in *The New Yorker.* Your dying is not really good news."

I don't know whether Jane could hear me, but hearing goes last. Hearing lasts longer, so she may have heard me. The oncologist came down that night, twelve hours before Jane died, and she said, "Jane knows I'm here." And doctors probably know more about this than I do. Then she said, "It will happen very soon."

Everybody was surprised it was quite so soon. But Jane was dying. So that night, I slept beside her. I slept in little snatches and woke up every twenty minutes to hear Cheyne-Stokes breathing going on. I was in bed with her living body. I knew it wouldn't be very long.

In the morning the breathing changed from the Cheyne-Stokes to the rapid little panting that signals the very end. The phone rang, right beside the bed, and I picked it up, looking at Jane. It was my daughter, and I said, "I think Jane just breathed her last breath." My daughter said, "I'll call back."

The next breath didn't come. I pulled Jane's eyelids down. Her eyes had been wide, not blinking for quite a while. She hadn't been seeing anything. I'd kept my body in front of her eyes just in case she saw me, but I don't think she did. She had died in her bed, in our bed. And that's what she had wanted.

It was Saturday morning, and the visiting nurse who was on duty was out of beeper range. Of course she had to come and certify that Jane was dead before the funeral parlor could come. Well, I'd told the funeral parlor, so they were ready. But I didn't want Jane's body to be brought out of the house. I just sat beside her dead body for about four hours. I talked to her. I touched her and felt her get cold. I wanted to be alone with her dead body. And I had four hours. I could have stood more, but finally the Visiting Nurse stopped by and then called up Chadwick's Funeral Parlor in New London and these people that she and I knew came with their gurney and a van in which they transport bodies.

I locked our dog, Gussie, up in my study. I didn't want him to see her go. He wouldn't have known anything, I suppose, but he searched for her forever. For the next year, he took her shoes constantly out from under the bed, and I wouldn't take them away from him. After about a year, he stopped. I don't, of course, know what he still thinks about her. Her smell will dissipate, the pheromones will break up. But her slippers were just with Gussie a tremendous amount of the time.

I felt by staying with her and feeling her get cold and kissing her cold lips that I'd know she was dead. But I think it took me a long time. Her body leaving the house was terrible. Two years later, her papers leaving the house was terrible, when the papers were being put into the archives. It took me two years to face the task of going through her things. Not being able to care for her any more was incredibly hard to face. There was nothing to do! Of course, the funeral gives you something to do. Fourteen hundred condolence letters gives you something to do. And I needed to deal with people to prepare the memorials to Jane and work on her book and read the book proofs—these are all connections to Jane.

At the time that Jane was actually dying, it didn't seem extraordinary to me that my daughter called just at that moment. My children called often. Other people were just holding their hands back from the dial. Because they knew. But my children knew I wanted them to call. They were a comfort. They weren't Jane's children. I was married before Jane. But they were permitted by their mother to love Jane, and I'm grateful for their doing that. They were magnificent in their attendance and care, all during her illness, and to me afterward. Every time I have a testimony of their love to me, I notice it a lot. I would not have minded if my daughter had stayed on the phone.

The progress of my grief was that for the first weeks, I couldn't think of anything except Jane's last few days. For months, almost a year, I could not see Jane with her hair on her head. She was bald, always. And finally I had a dream where she was in her beauty and she was naked in bed beside me and we were about to fuck, and I could see her still with hair. That was good. I mean it hasn't stayed the same. I just wrote a little thing the other day saying, more or less, "You think that their dying is the worst thing that can happen. Then they stay dead." For a year, I screamed. I wasn't depressed. I was outraged. I dreamed terrible nightmares.

People were enormously kind. In those fourteen hundred letters I got in the first month after her death, most of them were from people who didn't know us but who knew Jane's poetry. Her death got an awful lot of attention. It was even on NPR. "Fresh Air" rebroadcast an interview with Jane and me. People found out that way. *The New Yorker,* the week after she died, brought out three of her poems with her birth and death dates. A lot of people found out that way. So that's why so many letters came.

There were people who'd heard her read or had just read her poems and related to her because their husband was a depressive, or they'd met her for five minutes once, or they'd read the obit in *The New York Times,* the *Philadelphia Inquirer,* the *Los Angeles Times,* the *Boston Globe.* The obit even ran in a newspaper in Texas. The story was out on the wire. Some places picked it up. And every bit of attention to her pleased me.

There are some people who cannot talk about these things. In my case, I couldn't not talk about it; I couldn't stop talking about it. That's still quite a bit true. It's still quite true. It's curious. I was aware of this in my first year. I would do such things as—though this specific incident didn't really happen—go into a diner and the man next to me would say, "Can I have the ketchup?" and I'd say, "Here. My wife liked ketchup. She died of leukemia. She was forty-seven." You know, opening my heart to a stranger in an ancient diner. But I couldn't stop talking. Clearly some people wanted me to, but I couldn't stop. Now, after almost four years, when I am with somebody, Jane *always* comes up. Something about her illness and death comes up, almost always. I was dating a woman in New Hampshire. On the third date, she said, "Do you talk about Jane every date?" The woman wasn't being mean or sarcastic or anything. She was kind of curious. She was a nurse herself.

By this point, I talk about Jane more than I think about her. I think about her every day. But I'm more apt to start telling stories than I am to go into reverie and go over it and over it, which I did at first. Things do change.

I kept kissing Jane's lips after she died. I did when she was in the coffin, too. Everybody gets cremated. We didn't want cremation. We had bought our grave plot, in joy, shortly after we moved to New Hampshire, when we knew we would never go anywhere else and we could die there. We bought this grave plot so that we would be together. We used to walk there sometimes. We were a morbid lot!

I got the grave man, the monument man, to come over. I had had a notion of quoting some lines of poetry, but it was Galway Kinnell and his wife, Bobbie, who suggested the particular lines that are on our grave.

In the summer of '92, Jane had written a poem, another poem about my impending death, called "Afternoon at McDowell." I was on chemo and we went down to McDowell Colony when Richard Wilbur was getting the gold medal—because he is an old friend— and Jane talks about it in the poem and writes the line, "Thin after your second surgery." She always had a way of writing with apparent simplicity and making it into a complex structure that you feel but don't notice. The final stanza of the poem says, "After music and poetry, we walked to the car. I believe in the miracles of art, but what prodigy will keep you safe beside me?" And then the poem went on about my fumbling with the radio as we drove, looking for an inning of a Red Sox game.

So on her grave it says, "I believe in the miracles of art, but what prodigy will keep you safe beside me?" The stone has her name, Jane Kenyon, with two dates and it says Donald Hall with one date. And that's the prodigy. It's black granite, with white incisions. About two months after we stopped there, I suddenly realized that it looked like the Vietnam War Memorial, which we both loved.

I am very pleased with her grave. We walk down there in the graveyard, Gussie and I. "Augustus," Jane used to call him, "Augustus Tinkle Poop Wagtail IV." All these silly things couples make up! All through the house all the herbs have her handwriting. The house is a mess. Jane was not compulsively tidy, but she was tidier than I am. Beside the television is a huge pile of CDs and tapes, and just this spring, I noticed that behind them is a little electric grinder. I didn't put it there. It had to have been there for years. It says, "To grind Indian spices ONLY." I don't know why the grinder was there, why she happened to put it there. I can't imagine anybody else putting it there. But the note was in her handwriting.

All over the house, there are bits and pieces of her. It's better to live with bits and pieces of her than not to. But now I am able to go away to New York, taking just a few photographs with me. For the first few months, I couldn't leave the house overnight at all. I would have been leaving her. It was as if I was still her caregiver. That's all I can say. It just seemed a violation and I would be letting her down.

The one phenomenon that occurs to me, in terms of my grieving, is that I seem to feel that she got smaller and smaller, physically smaller. I had a dream, about a year after she died, that at the end of the room there were shelves, like bookshelving, but on them were a vast number—two hundred and fifty or so—little tiny bodies of Jane. And in my dream I said, "Oh, yeah. I've got to bury them. Yup. Yup."

One of the ways she becomes smaller is that she doesn't know about TWA 800. She doesn't know about Monica Lewinsky and Bill Clinton. So much she doesn't know, sometimes it makes me weep, seeing what she doesn't know. But that makes for a bit more distance. She has to be more distant.

After her death, I knew she was dead, in a way. There wasn't a supernatural sense of her being there. But the associations—the dog and the bed we slept in for all those years—these were all things that continued the closeness and the tie. Maybe it isn't that I wanted to continue to care for her or be her caregiver, but I wanted to stay close to everything that was hers, and ours.

Five months after her death I began to read poems again, publicly. I had done twenty-five readings a year for fifty years or so. But I couldn't do it while she was ill. I canceled everything. And then I couldn't do it at first after she died. But finally I got so that I could go away overnight, and it wasn't so bad. It only took me four years to be able to leave home and go to New York to teach for two and a half months. I couldn't have done that at first.

I don't think about my own death very much except when I smoke a cigarette. I certainly don't think about it as much as I used to. But I know I will be angry and scared if I find out I'm going to die. I remember Jane saying, "Dying is easy. But the separation is awful." I guess when it looked like I was dying, she felt that way. I don't think that ten years earlier that would have crossed her mind, that that was the worst thing that could happen—separation.

You think the dying is the worst thing. But that's something you can do something about, because you can scream your bloody head off or you can cry all the time. Four years later, though, the person you loved is still dead, and you can't do anything about it. That is the hardest part.

Julie Morton

I first met Julie Morton through her father, John, whose story I also collected during the years I interviewed people for this book. When I met Julie, she was a twenty-one-year-old college student whose mother, Mimi, had died earlier the same year after a heroic battle against a complex and prolonged series of illnesses. As a young adult, Julie faced the challenge of her mother's illness in part with the help of lessons she'd learned from a distant culture. She brought those lessons of community and unconditional love back to her New England home, to her dying mother and her grieving father. I was especially moved by Julie's innate wisdom, grace, and openness—qualities rarely achieved in only two decades of life but qualities that defined both Julie herself and her response to her mother's beautiful closing journey.

Before my mom was diagnosed with cancer, she had a blood-clotting problem. When I was six or seven, she had a miscarriage, followed by a blood clot in her leg. When I was about ten, she got a blood clot in her lung. My senior year in high school, she had a sinus infection that wouldn't go away. I knew that her situation was pretty serious, but I didn't really think about the possibility that her life could be in danger. She was in and out of the hospital, first with a bleed in her head and then with a clot. It was really easy for her to clot *and* bleed. It went back and forth.

With the sinus infection, she went into the hospital a couple of different times, but nothing really helped. At the time, I didn't think about death, even though people kept telling me that she was really close a couple of times. At that time, a lot of my friends wanted to get away from home. I was, instead, thinking about how important my family and my relationship with my mom were. We had always been close. Now, any little mother-daughter tensions seemed a lot less important, especially the ones in high school when you're at each other's throats.

My mom was diagnosed with cancer in November 1995. She didn't tell me right away. Even before I knew, though, I remember feeling "off" somehow, just kind of distracted. I had been thinking about her a lot and about generational patterns. My grandmother had died of cancer. I had heard theories that cancer has to do with issues of worth, of self-worth or self-love. I was noticing a lot of patterns that my mom had and that I would find myself repeating, like making sure that everybody else was okay all the time or putting myself down to make sure other people felt comfortable.

When I got home for Christmas break and learned about the cancer, I was angry that my parents had waited to tell me. I was shocked. I had known that cancer was a possibility because someone had said that her blood condition could develop into a cancer, but she had bone-marrow cancer—multiple myeloma—which was very rare. It is very rare in young people and in women. It's most common in the old. She wasn't a candidate, statistically.

My mom was in the hospital when I got home. She had had another bleed. Mom had a wonderful doctor who had worked with her since she had developed a blood clot in her leg. He told me that his mother had been diagnosed with breast cancer when he was in college. I remember him getting all choked up and telling me to take each day as a blessing and to appreciate whatever time we had together. Another doctor gave my mother six months to three years to live but said that some people lived fifteen years with this kind of cancer.

Our family policy was to be really positive and to say, "Hey, you can beat this." My mom was hard-core into the whole New-Age health craze: *Mind over body; you can visualize yourself out of anything.* She had been interested in health and healing for a long time. She was a massage therapist. After her cancer diagnosis, she bought Chinese herbs and did acupuncture and all sorts of visualization exercises. I felt comfortable with that approach because I was into that, too, from all of the things she and I had talked about and done. I remember thinking about the possibility of her dying, but I also remember thinking that you can't even give energy to the idea of death. I was convinced, right up until she died, that she was going to at least make it another five years.

Initially, my mom did okay. Everybody was surprised at how well she did. By that spring, she was doing really well. I went away during the following summer for a month and felt all right about doing that. Then in the fall, I went back to school. I thought she had the cancer under control. We even heard one of the doctors say something about remission, which turned out to be more rumor than fact. But we got excited about it. We considered doing a bone-marrow transplant, but she had only a 50 percent chance of surviving that because of her clotting problem. Basically, there isn't a whole lot of hope for people who don't do bone-marrow transplants for this cancer, but I thought that she was in remission. I really wanted to think that things were okay.

In the spring of my sophomore year, I again felt kind of weird. When I talked to my mother, she would minimize things a lot. She would say, "Oh, it's no problem. No big deal." I came home from school early and was really surprised at how sick she was. We had originally thought that all her health problems, one after the other, were separate and not connected to the cancer. She was in the hospital for pneumonia, and then she was in the hospital because she almost had kidney failure. It was one thing after the other.

In the summer, she had fevers, didn't feel well, and couldn't sleep. I stayed home and took two classes at a nearby college. I was feeling angry again. I really wanted to be there for her, but I was angry that I had to have this struggle going on in my life. I was even mad at my mother because on some level, I believed she could make herself better if she wanted to. Then I would be really upset at myself for having those feelings. It was awfully hard. I remember feeling, "Aren't we good enough? Don't we have an easy enough life or a good enough life that you can't just be happy and healthy where you are, right now?" In some ways I thought she wanted attention or something. I really didn't understand how much she was suffering.

As a result of my mom's illness, my dad and I became very close. We would go on "chill-out" walks every day and talk about what was going on and how we felt. Sometimes we would just kind of vent. We would often have a very similar perspective. It was wonderful for me to have him. I know how lucky I am in that.

In the fall, I went to Africa. I had talked to my mom about the trip; I had been wondering, When is *my* life going to start? I had spent all my free time away from school, at home. All my friends were going on trips across the country or going to work somewhere else, and I was just feeling, Oh, God. How long is this going to go on? When are you going to start to get better?

Mom had encouraged me to go to Africa because she knew how much it meant to me. The trip was a study-abroad program, through the School for International Training. My topic of study in Ghana was midwifery. I got to go north to work with a midwife in the town of Tamale. I was doing an independent study, so I was on my own. I got to hang out with these really cool women, and I got to be present at a birth, which was just amazing. The mother lived way out in the bush and had her baby right on the floor without all the white coats and machines and beeping things. It was an incredible, beautiful beginning.

The philosophy in Ghana is that when you have children, you are reincarnating your ancestors. It doesn't really matter how long you live or what you do so much as that you keep the cycle going. Everything is dying and being reborn all the time. For you to take part in that—to be part of that—is almost spiritual.

I thought about my mother constantly in Ghana. I would talk about what was happening with her because there was another girl on the trip whose father had died of brain cancer. I would think, That must be really tough. That's a possibility for me, but it's not going to happen. But as my time in Ghana progressed, I realized more and more that it could happen.

A lot of times in Ghana, when I was sick or tired, I would think, Oh, if I could just have some chicken soup that my mom made. My mom used to bring me soup when I was sick. She also would bring me honey-and-lemon tea. In Ghana, I'd think, I can't wait to go back home. I was still really wanting that mothering. I wasn't quite able to give that to my mom yet. I was still resentful. When I had tried giving it to her in the summer, I had been thinking, You should really be giving this to me, you know.

Every time I would call home, I would talk to my mom. I would call about once a week. I really had never been good at talking with my mom on the phone. We both always wanted to know what was going on with the other person. It was like "Oh, you'll hear about me. I just sent a letter off to you. Just tell me what's going on with you." My mom was minimizing stuff. When I left for Africa, the deal we had was that she would tell me if something was going on and if I was to come home. But I would talk with her on the phone; she would say, "Well, I'm taking steroids again," and I would think, Oh, steroids. Sure. I didn't understand that that was another way for her to say she was on chemotherapy again. But then I would get a letter from my dad saying, "She's back on chemotherapy, but things are okay. Things are okay."

I usually really enjoy being in new places, but my last week in Tamale and the last two weeks in Ghana were just miserable. In Tamale, the first thing people do is greet you. They greet you with "How did you sleep?" Then they say, "How's your mother? How's your baby?"—even though they don't have any idea what is going on in your life. And then, "How's your husband? How are you?" *Everybody* does that. When you greet people, you walk down the street and you do that. It made me feel, I need to be home. I had learned a whole new pattern for how I wanted family to be, where grandparents are really integral. I really wanted Mom to be alive for that, too. I had to wrestle a lot with the idea that she might not be around to see grandkids, which was just devastating to me. It still is.

I returned from Tamale to the southern city of Accra. All of a sudden I was back in a crowd, in a big city. When I called home from Accra, my dad answered the phone for the first time in months. He said, "You know Julie, Mimi had a reading with an astrologer." I think my mom had always been searching. My dad and I would joke about it. Another reading, I thought. Some other reading. Some other something. Oh, great.

My dad said Mom had asked the astrologer how long she had to live and asked if he could see anything significant in her chart. The astrologer said, "I see that you had cancer in your chart from the beginning. There's definitely cancer in here. And I don't see anything in your chart past April." This was the end of November. Then it hit me. I knew, if Dad was telling me this, that he didn't think she had very long, that he thought she was going to die, which was what I hadn't been able to think about at all.

Dad told me that Bobby, Mom's brother, had flown to see her from Denver and that when he saw her, he cried, my dad said, because she was so thin. I began to cry. In Ghana, you're not supposed to cry in public. If you cry in public, it means that something is just horrible. So people came over and said, "Oh it's not that bad. Don't cry."

In Ghana, I experienced a whole different way to care for people. Families are very, very important there. I learned how you can have a connection to someone else simply built on that person serving you. It was beautiful. Women in Ghana would take care of me. They would make me food. The women would argue to prevent me from helping to wash dishes. My host sister, who couldn't speak English, served me in a way that allowed us to become really good friends, even though she wouldn't let me serve her in return. My host sister knew how much I appreciated getting the food that she made. That kind of unconditional love was something I didn't know how to give my mom, but I was learning.

In the States, we're such an individualistic society that people think it's their right to not serve other people. It's not part of our culture to take care of our parents. We talk about the problems of "having to deal with our old people." You hear people say, "Oh, her mother *lives* with her. It's really a shame." In Ghana, an old people's home is a concept that is unthinkable, just unthinkable. And here I had been wondering, When is *my* life going to begin? When I got to Ghana, I realized, Oh, wait a minute. This *is* my life. This role is not so foreign. I can take a lot of joy in taking care of my mom.

I went home two weeks later. My dad picked me up at the airport in New York, and we drove home to New England. I was so psyched to see snow. It was so beautiful to me. We got back home and Mom wasn't awake. I thought, Oh? Usually my mom would be downstairs or she would even have come to the airport. We went upstairs to her room, and she was in bed asleep. We woke her up. She kind of rolled over and said, "Ohhh." She was sort of fuzzy. Then she said, "John, do you think you could make me a poached egg?" He said, "Oh, sure." This was after twelve hours of driving. He turned right around and went down and made a poached egg. To me, that symbolized how dire things were. Mom didn't ask how Ghana was. She didn't ask anything. Life was in a whole different focus.

In the days after I got home, I would see people and they would say, "How was Ghana? Are you in culture shock?" And I would think, I haven't even had time to feel that. I've just had to shift gears. I'm not even thinking about Ghana anymore.

I started making food when I got back, but Mom wasn't eating very much at all. She'd basically stopped eating. I kept forcing salads on her, saying, "You need to eat your greens." And finally she said, "Julie, why do I need to eat my greens? I don't have to eat my greens if I don't want to eat my greens." And I realized then, when she said that, that she had made a choice, and that was it. We didn't need to try to keep her strong. She didn't have to eat anything because she was going to die.

Mom wasn't sleeping through the night. I'd wake up in the middle of the night and hear her coughing. She had a violent cough. She would cough until she vomited. I would go in and rub her back, and it would calm her down. It was what Dad had been doing all fall.

The doctors still didn't know that all of Mom's problems were connected to the cancer. She still hadn't been told that, but she knew. She would have frequent nosebleeds and would cough herself sick. She would sit in her chair a lot and look out at the horizon, because we have such a beautiful view. When she talked to Jerry, the astrologer, it was incredibly helpful because he gave her permission to die, which a lot of us hadn't. He said, "Not only are you going to die, but it's part of your life's work." He said, "You can do this really well. You can die in a way that really affects a lot of people. You can make this a really beautiful transition for people, so they'll think about their lives and about death in a different way."

For Mom, all of a sudden, death changed from being a horrible, terrifying thing to something that was really a relief. She didn't have to think about all the shots she was going to get and all the treatments she had to go to. She wanted to die in a really conscious way, which was an incredible gift for Dad and me and for everybody else involved.

Before I had come back from Ghana, Mom had booked tickets and arranged to go to Germany so that she could see Mother Meera, an Indian saint who is supposed to be the Divine Incarnate, the Divine Mother. She's like the counterpart of *Si Baba,* who's also really big in India. I thought, Oh God, another one of these.

I don't even know how we got out of the house. My mom had a nosebleed. It was icing outside. The plane was canceled, but then officials decided to let it go anyway. Mom looked horrible. We got wheelchairs to move her around. I would just kind of hold her.

When we arrived in Germany, no wheelchair was ready for her. My dad went to find one. Mom was exhausted. We were both sitting there, and she lay down and put her head in my lap. I was holding onto her. I realized how frail she was. It was one of those moments: we both knew that we were together; we knew *that* moment was all we could count on. We sat there in the airport weeping, understanding how near physical separation we were.

We were to see Mother Meera for four sessions each week for two weeks in her living room. Dad and I were joking about bringing a novel or a Walkman to the sessions. Yet for me, the experience was profoundly moving. I felt it was Mom's way of bringing me to somebody who was a mother figure because she couldn't be that for me any more. It was almost a ritual pilgrimage so that I could say, "Okay, I release this. I give up my expectation that my mom might live." It was a way to say, "I'm giving up my control of this issue." It was a profound experience for me, simply in the act of making the trip. There we were, with no doctors' appointments, no people to update, no phones. Nobody knew where we were. It was just the three of us.

Sometimes it's hard to swallow that you are seeing an avatar. You throw that word around and get a lot of strange looks. This woman was pretty damn cool, though, whatever she was. People pack the room. Then Mother Meera, who's about thirty or thirty-five, comes in, eyes down, and sits down. Then everybody comes up to her, and she gives *darshan*. She holds each person's head for about ten seconds. You sit in front of her, and she holds your head, and then you sit back up and you look at her, and she looks into your eyes, and then you stand up and you walk back to your seat. It takes about three hours because there are tons and tons of people just *packed* into this place. Just the fact that she didn't say anything, just her presence, made me cry. I don't even know what was so powerful.

Day by day, Mom changed. She seemed to get much thinner. But she would have sundaes or ice cream—two times a day. It was like, Why not? After we got to Mother Meera's, I think she just let go. She was satisfied. An element of fear had been part of our lives for so long. There was always a "What if?" Now that element was gone because we *knew* the "What if." Now we knew that she was going to die, and in a way, she was almost having a good time with it. So she would eat her ice cream. It was funny because there were all these other people who would go to see Mother Meera, and Mom would say, "Well, I have cancer." And other people would say, "Are you coming for a cure?" She would say, "No, I think I'm ready to die." A lot of them couldn't handle that; from our cultural standpoint, the ultimate thing is to live. There were a couple of people there who were really supportive of her approach, but a lot of people said, "Have hope. You never know what will happen."

On the last day of that first week, my dad said, "There's no way she can do another week. I don't even think they're going to let her on the plane coming back if we stay here another week." Mom was not looking good. She wanted to go into the hospital in Germany to get some blood work done. My dad said, "If she goes into that hospital, they won't let her out." So he called Mother Meera's secretary and explained the situation. When the secretary told Mother Meera, she said, "Oh no, go home. You don't need to see me." Mom was fine with the idea of going home. We were both really surprised because she had been so determined to go over there. But now she said, "Okay. Four visits is good enough."

So we went home. In the plane, Mom was miserable. That was where I really felt I was mothering her. I had to change her clothes— she had long underwear on and was too hot. Then I had to give her her shot in the little tiny airplane bathroom. It was very surreal and strange. We arrived in Boston and Jerry, the astrologer, met us and drove us home. Mom was not doing well. She was exhausted and in pain. Dad had called her doctors from Germany to tell them that we were coming home and that we wanted to be able to come in to the hospital. He called the hospital the next morning, and her oncologist said that she would make a house visit instead. The next morning, her doctors came out to see her and took her off Heparin and gave her more morphine. It was really clear to me that we were coming upon the end if they took her off the blood thinner.

All of this time, Mom had been working on a letter to all of her friends to say she was dying and that she was okay with that. She wanted to tell them that they could write to her if they wanted but not to call. Seeing Mother Meera had done a huge amount for Mom's spiritual comfort. She was pretty satisfied and happy, especially when we stopped having to give her shots. She was black and blue all over from the shots.

Hospice brought a hospital bed to our home. A Visiting Nurse put an IV in her for morphine, so Mom didn't have to take it orally. It was snowing. It was beautiful out—all white. Dad and I kept going for our little walks. I remember feeling like time was passing very slowly. I was doing all the little caretaking things, like rubbing her back when she was coughing. I was trying really hard to just be with her, rather than trying to fix her. I was trying hard to understand. I wanted Mom to know that it was all right for her to die.

My mom loved to sing. She was really into singing during those last couple of days. One night just after we returned from Germany, some of her doctors came out to see her. Dad and I went for a walk to give them some time with her and also to take a break ourselves. When we returned, Mom had the doctors all in a circle around her bed, and they were all singing. They were singing and crying. For Mom, it was very important to die well, to be fully conscious of her dying and to let other people know that she was, and to have a good transition and a joyful one, too. It was really moving to see her doctors with her. It also was really beautiful to see her and my dad interact. She would just watch him walk around. I could tell that she was really grateful that he had gone with her to Germany because she knew how out of his element he was there. It was really painful for her to move. With bone-marrow cancer, your bones fracture easily. But she was pretty comfortable when she wasn't moving.

My dad and I were both able to cope. I think he has a defense mechanism from when his dad died when he little and from serving in Vietnam so that he can do what has to be done. We were both hanging in there. In a way, it was a relief to not be afraid of what was going to happen next, to just be. My mom was very frail and thin. Her skin was just stretched over her bones, but she was shining. I remember that. She was all eyes, but she just shone.

I believe that there is a spirit, and that it leaves the body. Hers seemed to leave bit by bit. She was almost more spirit than body by then. But she still was singing. She got to the point where she was making up songs. She would sing about dancing.

A couple of her friends came to visit, and she amazed them with her singing. She was very lighthearted about everything. She was getting so that she wasn't as clear about things. I don't know if it was the drugs or what. I was afraid that death might take a long time. Of course, now, it feels like it happened so quickly.

Then her sister, Sally, came with her little daughter, who was about ten. My mom was in a bad mood, sad and angry. The nurses said that when people get really close to death and stop taking as many breaths per minute as normal, they can have a panic attack. I think that was what happened. At first she wouldn't even look at us. She was just sitting in a chair and she wouldn't look at us. And then she looked at us and got really confused. Sally and I look similar, and for a second, I think my mom didn't know who I was. But then she worked it out, and she was really happy to see her sister. That was a final thing she had to take care of, to make that connection, to have Sally be there.

After the visit, Dad took Sally and her daughter to a motel for the night. I was sitting at the end of my mom's bed. She was looking out the window. On one side of her was a picture of Mother Meera. Outside, it was snowing. It was the outside view that held her attention. I was holding her feet. She said to me, "I'm sorry about this evening." She was quite incoherent. I said, "Did you think I was Sally?" She said, "Yeah, I think so. I don't know." I said, "That's okay." We were talking about, well, I was saying that it was okay for her to leave. I didn't want to hold her up. I felt like I was going to be the one who would keep her holding on. It was hard to say that to her, but I told her a couple of times because I wanted to make sure she knew. Every time I said it, it was hard. She started crying, and then she looked out the window. I was holding her feet and we stopped talking for a little while. And then she looked back at the picture of Mother Meera, and then she looked back out the window, and then she started laughing. And then she looked back at Mother Meera, and looked out the window. There were some birds out there. It was really clear to me at that point that even though I was there, the conversation had moved on. I felt like she was really good with wherever she was going. She was really in a different place.

The next morning, we had a conversation with the nurse about how to give the morphine and how to give shots through the IV to dry the fluid out of the lungs out so the death rattle isn't so loud. The other shot we had to give was Atavan. The nurse showed me how. Mom woke up and had a panic attack and the nurse kept saying, "What is it? Are you afraid of not having enough medicine? What are you afraid of?" Mom was crying. She was disoriented and looking around the room. The nurse was wonderful. Mom couldn't answer. Then the nurse said, "Are you afraid we're going to run out of medicine?" and Mom said, "Yes." The nurse said, "We won't. Don't worry. We have plenty."

Mom said, "I'm afraid of getting more shots." And the nurse said, "Don't worry. You're not going to get any more shots." Mom was still crying, distracted and upset. The nurse said, "Are you afraid of dying?" Mom said, "No. Well, no." Everything she said was in very small, fragmented sentences. Then Mom said, "I'm just on a journey." The nurse said to me, "This is a really good time to give her the Atavan. She's at peace. She's very calm. When she wakes up, she has fear, she has a panic attack, but you can prevent this pain." So I gave her the Atavan and then we went downstairs for lunch. That was the first time I saw the owl.

I hadn't realized that we would give Mom the Atavan and that would be it, that that would be the last time that she would be conscious. The nurse came back in the afternoon, and said, "Now is a good time to give her the next Atavan shot." I said, "Wait a minute. This is it, then?" The nurse said, "Yeah. She's very close now." It was terribly hard for me to be the one giving her the Atavan. I was really afraid that I was making a decision for her, that that was the last time she would be able to talk, and that I had chosen that time. That night, the nurse and I both slept in the living room, next to her bed, and every four hours, I'd give her an Atavan shot.

That night, Dad and I sat with Mom for a while, and we sang songs that she liked. We sang, "How Could Anyone Ever Tell You?" and some lullabies that I remembered from when I was little. We sang "Michael, Row Your Boat Ashore," "The River," and "Wanting Memories," by Sweet Honey In The Rock, which was her favorite song. We sang for an hour or two. Eventually we both fell asleep, but then we woke up because her breathing was getting really, really heavy.

All through this time, we'd been playing George Winston's music. When we woke up, we could tell her breathing was more labored. For the last few days, she would breathe, and we would wait for the next breath. Sometimes Dad and I would be there together, and we would look at each other intently, and then she would breathe again. That night, she looked like she wasn't there at all. You could see the whites of her eyes. Her eyes were mostly rolled back. Her lids were half open. Her mouth was open when she breathed, and there was no flesh on her, no fat, just skin and bones. Her breathing became more and more labored. We could hear her lungs filling up with fluid.

We put on some Indian music that she had really liked. You know the mantra *Ohm namshi via. Ohm namshi via.* It's a song that she had listened to a lot to relax. We had read somewhere that it's a really good thing to die with God's name, in whatever language it is in—a name for the Divine—in mind. So you can help that by having it playing.

We lit a candle. We sat there and held her hand for a couple of hours. I don't even know how much time it took. Her breath was really labored; then all of a sudden it became easier and easier, more and more shallow. She took fewer breaths. She became quieter and quieter, and Dad looked up at me and raised his eyebrows. I guess he had been watching her pulse, and it had just stopped. I wouldn't have been able to tell you the moment she died, because it was so calm.

We just sat there for a little bit and cried. At the same time, it was a huge release. It felt like she had done what she wanted, and she'd done it really well. So we went downstairs and made tea and got out a family photo album and started looking through it. Before I went to bed for some sleep that morning, the sky was just incredible, with beautiful magenta streaks all the way across it. When I saw it, I remembered my grandmother talking about the sky the morning her mother died and how amazing it was. And when my grandmother died, my mother said the same thing had happened to her. It was odd because I had forgotten those stories until I saw a similar beautiful sky that morning.

Before my mother died, I couldn't ever think past that event, even when I knew she was going to die, even as far as where we would live or what we would do. I couldn't even imagine. I still feel like death is one moment that stops—*everything*. It's a cutoff point. But the memorial service was a sort of celebration. All of my high school singing group friends came and sang "Wanting Memories." Our point was to celebrate her life and her joy in living.

In the next few weeks, I saw the owls a lot. They were a personal thing for me. When I first saw the owl, the time I first gave my mom Atavan, I thought, What is this? I thought of the Native American interpretation that an owl sometimes symbolizes death or a transition. I *never* see owls around here—and this was in broad daylight—but there was an owl. And then two days after she died, there was another owl. After that, I saw lots of them. I was driving and I saw two owls. Then I saw lots more of them, probably around twelve owls in all, over the space of about two weeks. I haven't seen one since then.

But I couldn't figure it out. I thought, What is the deal with these owls? I even have a little rose quartz owl that my mom and I used to exchange when I would go away on a trip. We started doing that when I was in junior high school. I can't remember whose owl it was originally. I would leave the owl with her, and she would give me something in return, sort of as little tokens, for love. I could hold it and think of her. When I went to Ghana, I brought that rose quartz owl with me. When I went anywhere, whenever I would go away, I would bring it.

I also saw an owl one day when I was driving along, all upset. I actually was thinking that I had worms from Ghana. I didn't end up having worms, but that was my concern. I had to have something to worry about! I was thinking about maybe going into the hospital. I was driving along where there's never a cop, ever. I was tearing it up, going really fast. And there was this owl, *right* over the road. There was a branch and on it there was an owl. I slowed way down, and I looked up and I thought, What is the deal with this owl? I just don't get it. I drove right around the curve and there was this cop car and I thought, Huh.

I still haven't fully realized that my mother is gone. In those months that followed, I was in a fog. I didn't comprehend her death as being final, at all. I had been wrapped up in trying to take care of her, trying to rub her back or get her from the hospital to wherever—all those little mundane things that you can focus on so that you don't have to deal with the emotional enormity of the situation. My mom was my best friend in a lot of ways because I had a lot of time to get to know her.

The sense of loss seems to come in waves. But I feel like the journey with my mom was a gift because I've learned a lot. It has encouraged me to have a whole new connection with my spirituality that I really wouldn't have had to rely on or deal with or look at. I feel extremely privileged to have had the opportunity to have talked about death with my mother and to have intimately been with her at her death. Being present at death enriches you because—like the Ghanaian philosophy—all those parts of life are important, even the pain and suffering and sorrow and loss. It's loss, but it's also a celebration. I'm really lucky to have had her as long as I did. I'm lucky that she was so open about how she wanted to die and that I was able to be there. Intellectually, I know that my mom died very well, in a beautiful way. Emotionally, I have to allow myself to grieve, too, which has been a challenge. It's hard for me to balance all that out sometimes.

We create structures to allow our world to make sense to us. Yet so many things happen that are beyond our control, beyond our comprehension. My mom's passing was a beautiful illustration of that. When she died, she was illuminated by something. It was clear to me that she was passing into something extraordinary.

If we are able to be more present in these transitions, then we might be able to take some of the fear out of them. It's not something that we talk about often in our culture. I have difficulty talking about separations like death sometimes because it is so emotionally charged that it often brings up all sorts of issues for the person with whom I'm talking. But I feel that the more we're able to talk about things like death, the more it's discussed and addressed and the more differing perspectives that can be shared, then the more people are able to think deeply about death and finally, to accept it.

Tim Palmer

At the time that Tim Palmer shared the following story with me, he was working as the executive director of Vermont CARES, an AIDS service organization. His partner, Scott, had died of AIDS a decade earlier. I learned about Tim through my daughter, Emily, who was working at the time as an Ameri-Corps*VISTA volunteer at Vermont CARES. Emily had often spoken to me about Tim's leadership skills and his sensitivity and insight as the director of a small nonprofit battling one of the greatest plagues ever to hit the human race. When I had the privilege of sitting with Tim and listening to him talk about Scott, I felt that I was bearing witness to a story of the greatest respect and love that two people can have for one another, both throughout their lives and into death.

I don't know where most of us learn how to do it, how to be with someone when he dies. It's all firsthand experience, because there isn't anything else like it. There isn't a tool to help you say, "Other people have walked this path before me. There is a path here and all we have to do is just try to find it."

When Scott and I first met, he was a student at Albany Law School and I was working in the State Legislature. We met in the state capitol building because he was doing an internship at the state Office of Court Administration. Our meeting was as a result of a bill in which he was very interested. There was no magic in that conversation. We met again about three months later at a bar. We were so different. He was intelligent, articulate, outgoing, funny, and attractive. He was a person to whom others felt drawn. I've grown a lot since our relationship, but at that point I was very quiet and isolated. I was intelligent, but I really was not fully who I am now. One of the great gifts of our relationship was that we constantly challenged each other to see who we were and who we could be.

That first night in the bar, we spent most the time just talking. I invited him over for dinner a week later, and we spent that evening talking. Scott admitted several months later that it was the first time that a relationship had started like that. In so many gay relationships, if there is physical attraction, there is the immediate physical gratification. Scott realized that this was going to be something different.

Shortly after we started seeing each other, Scott graduated from law school and had to move to Elmira. He had a year's internship in a court in Chemung County. We were physically separated for a year, so we did the long-distance commute. After that year, he moved back to Albany and we moved in together. From that point on, for thirteen years, we were together, and every day of those thirteen years was an adventure.

Scott had a large core group of friends with whom he spent a great deal of time. In contrast, I always had a very small, intensive group of friendships. Even the way we interacted with other people changed over the course of our relationship. Scott increasingly became focused on individual friendships, and I learned to broaden into a larger circle of friends. As a couple, we developed a group of about thirty friends with whom we would spend evenings or even take vacations.

Scott always liked to do things on the spur of the moment. I have to plan forever! He would come home on Thursday night and say, "Do you want to pack some clothes?" I was the packer. He hated to pack, so I would pack for both of us. And I would say, "You want to tell me for what?" And he would say, "Don't worry. I've already called your office. You have tomorrow off and you have Monday off. We're going to get on a plane." And I'd say, "You have to tell me something. I need to know what to pack." So he would just give a description: It's going to be warm or cold, or we're going to be able to go to a beach. He would only give that much information. I would usually be in the air before I would even know where we were going.

Scott was diagnosed with HIV on Presidents' Day weekend in 1989. Before that, he had refused to be tested because at that time there was really no viable treatment. And he felt that he wanted to live every day without thinking about his own mortality. After he was diagnosed we thought back to a very serious illness he had had about eight years earlier. That's when we think he was first infected. Studies have shown that right after infection, many people develop a flulike illness. Scott had been very sick then for two weeks. The doctors couldn't figure it out. They kept saying, "It's the flu, the flu." So we went on with our lives.

On that Presidents' Day weekend, Scott was having a great deal of difficulty breathing. We went to the hospital. It turned out he had PCP. He was admitted. The doctor came in and said, "You have pneumonia. Do you want us to do other tests?" Scott said, "Well, I guess I know the results of what one of those tests would be." And the doctor said, "I think we're pretty safe in assuming that you do." It turned out that Scott also had the beginning of Kaposi's sarcoma. He also had another infection, another viral infection.

We were at Albany Medical Center, and we were together in his room. Scott had been in the hospital now for a couple of days. A doctor was doing grand rounds with about half a dozen students. The doctor stood outside of Scott's room in the hospital, and said, "This is a thirty-five-year-old, gay white man who has three opportunistic infections. He had not been tested before he came to the hospital a few days ago. His prognosis is not good. He will likely be dead within two or three weeks."

Up to this point, the doctors had never had a conversation with Scott about their prognosis. They hadn't had one with me, either. I walked out of the room and grabbed the physician's arm and said, "You're coming with me." He said, "Excuse me?" I said, "You're coming with me!" He said, "I'm doing grand rounds." I said, "Do you want me to correct you in front of the students or not? It's up to you." He said, "Well, could this wait?" And I said, "No, this can't wait. And since you are refusing to, I will do it in front of the students. Maybe this is a lesson they should have.

"Don't you *ever* stand outside a patient's room and have the kind of conversation you just had. Do you know that neither the patient nor I have ever been told by any physician on this staff what his prognosis was? Do you have any idea what you could have done to his ability to improve? But if you knew Scott, you'd know that you have probably improved his chances of surviving because he's going to prove you wrong! But don't you ever, ever do that outside of another patient's room."

The physician said, "How dare you!" I said, "How dare *I?*" He said, "You shouldn't correct me in front of the students." I said, "You wouldn't come with me. I'm done with you. You're not permitted to come into Scott's room. You're not permitted to have any students come into his room. We are not part of your grand rounds. And I don't want to see you. I don't want to hear from you. I don't want to have you involved in Scott's care in any shape, form, or manner. You are now excused. You may go."

He walked away with the students. The head of the AIDS unit visited about an hour later and apologized profusely. I said, "Why weren't we told? Why did we have to hear it this way?" And he said, "We were planning on coming in and talking with you." I said, "Scott is an intelligent person. He hasn't lost his mental capacities. He's quite capable of taking news like this." He said, "We were just concerned that you've been hit by so much in such a short period of time that we didn't want to share that information with you that quickly."

I said, "Rule number one, in dealing with Scott, and I would suggest with other patients, is that you get a sense of who they are. You need to know that Scott is a person who likes to know everything as soon as it's known. He doesn't like people knowing things about him that he doesn't know. Don't try to protect him. Give him all the information you have."

From that point on, the relationship with the physicians was great. They were very forthcoming and direct and honest. They wanted to get him on clinical trials and all kinds of things. Scott really put them through their paces.

One day I was visiting Scott in the hospital, and a person who worked in the New York State Senate walked by the room. It was about four or five days after Scott had been admitted. Scott had not had a conversation with his own employer when this person walked by and saw us. The man physically reacted, paused, then kept walking.

I went out to the hallway. The man had already left the unit, and I couldn't find him in the hospital. So I called and left a message on his home machine saying, "I know that you saw us in the room. But I don't want you to draw any conclusions, and I don't want you to have a conversation with anyone until you have a conversation with me. And I intend to be at your office tomorrow morning to have this conversation." I showed up at the guy's office the following morning. His receptionist said to me, "I'm really sorry." I said, "What are you sorry about?" She said, "I heard about Scott." I said, "How did you hear about Scott, and what did you hear?"

She said, "I heard he's in the AIDS unit." And I said, "I don't know what you may have heard or what you think you may know, but where Scott is, is his business. I do not want you talking to anybody about this rumor, and if you have already spread it, I want you to tell people with whom you have shared this gossip that that is all it is and that they should not spread it. If I hear from anyone in these halls—and I travel them quite often—if I hear from anyone that they know where Scott is or that they're sorry that Scott is at the AIDS unit, or anything like that, I will come back at you, and I will do it in such a way that you will regret ever having said anything about Scott."

Then I went in and talked to her boss. I made it very clear to him that his violation of Scott's privacy was something that wasn't acceptable, that he had a responsibility because he was at the wrong place at the wrong time, and that he had to hold that information as private until Scott had the opportunity to disclose whatever he wanted to disclose to the people who meant the most to him in the legislature.

The legislator and his secretary did maintain the secret.

Eventually, Scott decided to leave his job. He felt that he needed to focus on working with other people living with the virus. He was one of those people who believed that if he wasn't working 300 percent, he wasn't working. But he took the summer of '89 off. It was then that we got our dog, actually *his* dog. The two of them became totally inseparable and insufferable. And he also spent that summer working in our gardens with other people who were living with the virus. Scott was a great gardener. And he was also doing some writing. He was working on a very funny comedy-club routine. And we traveled a lot.

Scott had always wanted to go to the northwest coast, the Seattle area. He'd never been there. So we went. He'd always wanted to go to Disneyland. It wasn't number one on my list, but we went. We got to visit a number of friends who were also sick. It was the summer of closure for him. It was a time for him to start new things, finish up others, and contemplate his future. We didn't know how long he would have.

I was working at that time. I was spending a lot of time with Scott going to clinic and going on these trips. It gave me the opportunity to be closer to him. And in the midst of it, it was overwhelming. The world that we had so safely constructed was collapsing, but many new things were coming out of it. We were letting go of knowing that we would be together for fifty years; we were recognizing that we had this opportunity now and that it would not go on forever.

One day, when Scott was not doing particularly well, we were taking a ride and he started crying. I said, "What's the matter?" And he said, "I fear that when I'm gone, you're not just going to get on an airplane and do something. You're going to lose that ability." And I said, "I have a surprise for you. I've already packed. We're not just going out for a ride. We're going to the airport." I think that was the day he really realized how immense an impact he'd had on my life.

When you're born gay, you spend the first eight years of your life like everybody else, doing all the fun things. And then you start recognizing that you are different. Because you're different, you start seeing things slightly askew from the way your friends might see them. The struggle of coming out is really over the fact that we're all socialized into wanting the spouse and two children and the picket fence and the nice house, and you realize—I realized when I was coming out, unlike today—that what you believed can't be possible. You can't have that kind of singular relationship. You can't have a family.

When you're gay, when you're first coming out, you don't think in terms of, I will always be somebody's partner. You don't think that's possible. I think what that summer with Scott did for me was move that coming-out process to a whole new level of awareness. Here I was, one more time being challenged to believe that while all of those things are great, that's really not what my life was about.

I think the hardest part of it was seeing so many things opening up. It was like a springtime, to see so many things, internally and in the relationship, opening up and yet to know that it wasn't likely that we would get to harvest them. Scott was my best friend. Even in the midst of having Scott deal with the physical and mental realities, I had the opportunity to share with him what I was going through, and he was there for me. He was there, but I knew that the point would come when I would go through what I thought was going to be the most difficult period, and Scott wouldn't be there.

It was wonderful to watch Scott do things he'd never done, to spend time with people that he loved, and to make a difference in many people's lives with the work that he was doing. It was one of those three-month periods where you say, "If I didn't know what was driving this, this would be the most wonderful time anyone could possibly have." Unfortunately, it *was* the illness that was driving us. I wish we could have that knowledge all of our lives so that instead of three months we would have seventy years of being open to people and opportunities, open to who we are, not afraid to say yes, not afraid to say no. I am terribly conflicted when I talk about these periods, about how wonderful they were and how horrible they were at the same time.

After that Presidents' Day weekend, Scott was hospitalized three more times in 1989, once in the summer and twice in the fall. The hospitalizations were getting shorter. They were basically to deal with the Kaposi's sarcoma. The doctors wanted to put him on clinical trials for the new cancer treatment for Kaposi's. He struggled with that. I think he was in denial about Kaposi's. He felt he'd beaten PCP, he'd beaten that other infection, and Kaposi's was the only thing he couldn't beat. The treatments were experimental, but he had ultimately decided to try them. He did them not for the purpose of improving the quality of his life, because they didn't. They did just the opposite. But he figured, If doctors can learn something from me, and I'm this close to the end, well, then let them learn something. And they did. They learned not to use the dosage they used.

In the fall, he decided that he wanted to go back to work. I wanted to give up the lobbying piece of my job, so Scott took that on. We went to work together, for the first time. We had always worked very closely with each other in the same general field, but this was the first time that we actually worked together. He was in the office, and it was great fun. The staff there fell head over heels in love with him. That fall, he helped everybody involved in the organization focus on the things that were important. He also got them to have fun, which I'm not very good at doing. Then in January, when the legislature started, he was over there on a regular basis.

He had the freedom of knowing that this likely would be his last legislative session. You know how people in the legislature show up in somber gray suits, with all the charts and graphs and such? Well, Scott started showing up in a gray suit but in a very different tie or shirt combination. He would testify without papers, without written testimony. He used no charts or graphs. He would just talk about the issues. In New York, the legislature is very bureaucratic. People take themselves very seriously. And so for them, this was totally out of the natural realm of things. To have somebody who had spent eight years working as a staff member, to have this person show up and not follow the rules, was quite shocking to them. Everybody wanted him to testify on everything.

Scott and I would testify on housing and health care and economic development and education and roads and bridges. We would cover the waterfront because there was no one else advocating for the rural communities. As the session progressed, Scott became increasingly rural, going back to his roots. He would show up in jeans.

On Memorial Day weekend of 1990, Scott had just started the cancer treatment for the Kaposi's, and he became very, very ill. Scott's very good law-school friend, Mary Ann, and her husband, John, and their new baby, Madison, came over for a Memorial Day picnic. Scott had been getting progressively sicker because of the medication. He was supposed to go back in the hospital the night of

Memorial Day for another round of treatment. We had an amazing day with Mary Ann, John, and Madison. It was the longest time Scott had spent with Madison, who was, I think, just three months old. Her baptism was supposed to be the next weekend. It got into the evening and I said to Scott, "You're supposed to go in to the hospital. Do you want to?" He said, "No. I'm not going."

Instead, he went to work the next day, on Monday. He had been progressively getting more and more ill. He started out that day vomiting. He didn't have any control over his bladder at that point either.

When John and Mary Ann got over there in the afternoon, he had rallied. It was one of those windows of good health. He was well enough to go in to work the next day. He actually testified that day at one of the hearings. That night, when we got home, he said, "I think we should go to the hospital." So we went in. They gave him the cancer treatment, and Thursday they released him and he came home. He got very, very ill that night.

Two of his other law-school friends were coming up to visit him the next day. He didn't want them to have to visit him in the hospital. He wanted to be home. So I stayed with him that morning. They got there around noon. I wanted to give them some space. One of them was actually his first love, and it was great to see Scott's reaction to their being there. It was also great to be able to walk away for a while and just say, "He's with two people who love him, and if something happens, it happens, and it happens with people who care."

At about 3:00, one of them called me at work and said, "We've just called the ambulance. Scott is extremely ill, and neither of us knows what to do, so we've called the ambulance and we're going to take him to the hospital." I said, "Okay, I'll meet you there." I knew that the end had to be pretty close, but I didn't have any idea how close it actually was. When I got to the hospital, they had already arrived. The doctor met me and said, "I don't think he's going to make it through the night."

I had gone to all of Scott's clinic visits. I had been there when he was making the decision to go through the clinical trials. I'd been there for the decision of the do-not-resuscitate order and all that. As a lawyer, he had made sure that I had medical power of attorney and all of those sorts of things. He was very careful about all of those details. He had wanted me as his partner every step of the way.

When I went in to see Scott, I asked how he was doing and he said, "Well, you know how I'm doing." And I said, "Yeah, do you know?" And he said, "I've had better days." I said, "Yes, you have." And I told him what the doctor had said. He said, "I don't think so." I said, "Well, you're more in control of that than the doctor is, aren't you?" He said, "Yeah." So he made it through the night.

Our friends had to go back to New Jersey. Mary Ann came over and spent a really long time with him that night. And another group of friends was coming up from the city for that weekend for Mary Ann's daughter's baptism. On Saturday, we had a constant flow of people visiting Scott from law school and college. It was the first time I had met some of them. For those I knew, it was great to see them again and to watch them deal with Scott and with their own feelings about Scott and about death.

So I spent more time out of the room that day, with various friends of his in the halls or in the cafeteria, just talking to them. Scott and I had talked about this many, many times. I knew that he was in control of what he was in control of, and nobody was going to say he had to do this, that, or the other thing. I could see, watching him, that he was closing down. He was helping his friends find closure. It was almost like an assembly line. Mary Ann would talk to them before they went in to see Scott, to prepare them, because he was physically very different looking from what they were used to. He was unbelievably thin. Scott had always been big, robust, full of life. So Mary Ann did all the prep work. Friends would go in and see him. Then Scott would talk them through the situation. Then I would get them at the other end and would help talk to them about what it had been like over the last eighteen months, and I would tell them things like how important the card was that they had sent.

I spent that day helping other people deal with what they were feeling and telling them it was okay, telling them, "I don't know exactly what you're feeling, but whatever it is, it's okay. You don't have to feel sorry at this point. You don't have to feel angry. Whatever it is you're feeling, go with that one."

That night, Scott was better. So I stayed, and Mary Ann went home. The baptism was going to be on Sunday. Sunday morning, I ran home to get something ready for the baptism and Scott called me and asked where I was and what I was doing. He said, "Have I gotten anything in the mail?" Over the last couple of weeks, Scott had fallen in love with catalogues, 800 numbers, and his credit card. This was late May, early June, and he was planning his garden and ordering shrubs and trees. He also was ordering clothes because he was planning his summer vacation. Since things were arriving every day at the house, Scott asked if a particular delivery had come from a clothing store and I said, "Yes." He said, "Could you bring it in?" and I said, "Where do you think you're going?"

He said, "After the baptism, Mary Ann promised to bring Madison over, and she is going to take me on a ride through the hospital. I don't think I should go naked, do you?" And I said, "No, I don't think that would be good, but you do have a hospital gown." And he said, "And the difference between a hospital gown and naked is *what?*" I said, "Okay, good point." And so I brought in the new clothes, and I was putting them in the little drawer in the room and Scott said, "What are you putting them away for?" And I said, "It's going to be a few hours before Mary Ann gets here with the baby." He said, "I can't wear them now?" He was hooked up to his tubes and everything, but we changed him into the new clothes, the nurse and I. We had to get him all propped up in the wheelchair. John and Mary Ann called and said, "We're on our way. He should be ready."

Scott was very weak at that point, so we had to use a lot of pillows. He was terribly fragile. We had to be very careful in lifting him. At that point, he was basically skin and bones. There were very few muscles left. The medication had really debilitated him very quickly. It was a very, very high dose, which was what they learned about the dosage, that it was too much.

Dressing him that time was the moment that I knew that it was going to be over. The doctors' previous warnings had concerned me, but trying to dress Scott that day was physical reality. I was really seeing him struggle to do things that even when he was the most sick, he didn't have trouble doing. His body was in such sharp contrast to the brightly colored summer clothes in which we were putting him. He never liked being taken care of, so there was also resistance on his part. He would notice another Kaposi's sarcoma lesion. They were just sprouting at this point. He would joke about it, saying, "Oh, five more!" And then other times he would just be very, very depressed by it. He was focusing on being able to hold Madison and have Madison ride in the wheelchair with him. But there were moments when he would go from that really funny kind of storytelling or joking with a nurse or debating my wisdom to complete tenderness toward me.

He said, "I hope Madison remembers this ride." The nurse helped somewhat, but we were alone a lot during this process of getting dressed.

Scott had had two absolute rules that he had told me on Presidents' Day weekend in 1989. He said, "There are two things that I will not permit to happen. First, I will not have a lesion on my face. Second, I will not lose my mental capacities." And I said to myself, "Okay, if anyone can do it, it will be Scott." But the morning of the ride with Madison, Scott discovered the first lesion on his face. We talked about it. He was angry that he hadn't been able to prevent it, and I think he was angry that he hadn't died before it happened. It was also, for him, after the great day on Saturday when he had watched and helped lots of very close friends of his deal with his mortality, it was like, Okay, I'm not helping others deal with it any more. It's now time for me to be closer to this. While Scott was very open about the fact that he was dying, I think we all have to keep a little bit of that denial in us, and to use it effectively to maintain that distance. He was talking now about this being the right time to let go.

So Scott and Madison had their ride together in the wheelchair. I stayed in the room just to clean up. They were gone for an hour and a half. They visited every ward. I heard about it for weeks afterward. Different nurses and doctors and other people would say, "Well, we did see Scott that last day and he was still Scott." Even on that last day, he was funny and engaging and warm.

When they got back, after that long a trip, he was really tired. Mary Ann and I quickly changed him back into his hospital gown. He said about his new clothes, "I don't want to get these dirty. I want to make sure they're ready for my summer vacation."

Mary Ann said that during the walk Scott had engaged everyone in conversation, in the hallways, in the elevators, everywhere. He was holding Madison, and Madison was a perfect angel the whole time. She was focused on Scott's voice and the colors of his shirt. Scott just held her. Scott was the youngest of four children, so he had never been around a baby. Because Scott and Mary Ann's family were so close, Scott saw Madison as "my chance to have a baby." So while he was entertaining the world, he was focused on the baby. And the baby was focused on him. Mary Ann said that they stopped in the cafeteria so that Scott could get a milkshake. He couldn't keep anything down, but he wanted his milkshakes. And they just sat there. A group of nurses and doctors came over to see the baby and to see Scott, and they sat there for half an hour, all those people. He regaled them with stories, and Mary Ann said it was like last weekend when we were all together. It was like having Scott back. He was just *on* the entire time.

So we got him into bed, and Mary Ann and John and Madison went home. That night the Tonys were on. As part of that summer and fall of doing whatever it was that we wanted to do, we had seen *all* of the shows that were nominated for a Tony.

Just before the Tonys began, Scott's brother, Tom, called. Scott and Tom were talking, and Scott hung up right in the middle of the conversation. I knew it was in the middle of the conversation. He just hung up, and I left the phone on the bed, thinking his brother would call back. Scott at that point rolled over and fell asleep for a while. And then he woke up, maybe five or ten minutes later, and said, "What's the phone on the bed for?" And I said, "I was thinking that Tom might call back." And Scott looked at me with this look of "Who's Tom?" And then we just sat there. After thirteen years, we were able to read each other pretty well. From the look he gave me, I knew that this was it. He had broken one rule in the morning, and now the second rule was being broken in spite of his determination.

The two of us were alone. I climbed into the hospital bed with him, and we watched the Tonys. Every category that came up, we would debate who was going to win. Scott was fully engaged and thoughtful, but his breathing became more and more shallow. The nurse came in several times and did vitals. His pulse was dropping.

He stayed alert, but he slipped in and out throughout the entire ceremony. When the show was over, I turned the television off. Scott just lay there and looked at me and smiled and said, "Wasn't that great?" I said, "Yeah." He said, "It's been a great ride." I said, "Yes, but we still have a distance to go." And he said, "Yeah, but you won't have to buy a seat for me." I said, "No, I probably won't." And so we just lay there and I said, "Do you want me to get the nurse?" Scott said, "No. This is the way I want it to be. I don't want anyone here but you."

I said, "Well, then that's the way it will be." He started breathing in an increasingly gasping kind of breath. We were just lying there. He kept pressing against me, wanting to get closer. I had my arms around him. We were lying basically side by side, with his head on my shoulder. He started to burrow. Then he looked up at me and said, "I've got to go."

So I held him closer. It was three more breaths after that. Being there, holding him, I felt this life force that was Scott just dispersing. At the point of his last breath, I don't know how to describe it. I've actually never described it to anybody. I just felt as though that physical struggle was over. It was so peaceful a transition that there was just a sense on my part that he had willed it, that—as he was telling me when he shot me that look earlier in the evening—this was the way he wanted it, and that what he was basically doing in this physical struggle was simply letting go.

Part of why he wanted to be so close in those final minutes is that he needed assurance, that last physical touch, so that he could let go of the physical. The way I've thought about it is that he was as close to another human being as a baby in its mother's womb. This is at the other end of life. You need to be connected to another human being at that point.

There was this sense that had been building over the previous two days, with all the friends who visited, of just a dispersion of Scott's life force. Everybody who had walked out of that room had walked out with something they hadn't had when they walked in. Intellectually, I watched it. I knew it was happening. But I didn't want him to die. You can know that it's happening, intellectually, but it's a very different thing to be there at the end. That's when everything came together for me, and I think Scott knew that. I think that he needed to know that I was okay.

We had talked, Mary Ann, Scott, and I, about a month beforehand about assisting him in ending his life. My initial reaction had been, "I can't do that." Since then, I've assisted several other friends, but that was the first time I was faced with that possibility, and I wasn't ready. It was the one time in the entire eighteen months where I said, "I can't. I'll do anything that you want me to do, but I can't do that one."

Scott knew that I was struggling with it. He needed that last four hours just to get the sense from me that it was okay, that I was there, that I not only intellectually knew what had happened the day before but that I *emotionally* knew what had happened the day before, with all the friends. I think that's what he meant, at the end, when he said, "Wasn't that great?" and when he talked about it being a pretty good ride. He was basically asking permission to go.

Throughout the last eighteen months of Scott's life, in particular, and the last week and the last weekend and the last day, I became increasingly aware of how I was changing spiritually. I was raised a very strict Irish Catholic; I feared death. I feared anything approaching death. I had the construct of heaven and hell and all that other stuff. Scott had been raised a Methodist and didn't have any of those "problems."

Now, because of this experience with Scott, I don't fear death at all. I fear being afraid of it. I fear being at the end and not being able to embrace it. But that fear is almost gone, too, because of my own experience, not only with Scott but also with so many other friends—watching them embrace it—watching some friends struggle against death and others embrace it. Believe me, having seen so many other people die, when my time comes, I don't want to fight. I want to go. Whatever that transition is, however that happens, I know that while I physically won't be here any more, I know that in other people's voices, in other people's thoughts, in other people's ways of looking at things, there will be my voice, my thoughts, my way of looking at things, integrated into who they are. Not a day goes by that I don't hear Scott responding to something crazy or listening to music in the way that close friend had once helped me learn. Now there are things that I hear in music that I never would have heard before, but for that relationship and that friendship.

Scott continues to have a huge impact on my life. I realize that I am who I am as a result of the shared experience, the highs and the lows of a relationship with a person who was truly my soul mate. I don't know that we all get the opportunity to find that person, but I did.

Scott always used to keep a list of people to whom he had sent Christmas cards. The list also indicated whether he had gotten a card from them. He kept the list in a bound journal. It's the only thing that he was ever really organized about. That's another way in which we were very different. I have a tendency to be very organized, and if Scott could find a piece of paper five minutes after had written on it, it was a miracle.

In 1993, I was working in Boston. I was about to do my holiday cards, and I pulled out Scott's journal. I had kept it up for the three years after he had died. For some strange reason, in 1983, Scott apparently hadn't been able to find his journal, so he had kept the card list on regular sheets of paper. When he was done, he found the journal and stuck those sheets of paper inside. In 1993, they fell out of the journal as I was pulling it out of the bookshelf. I foolishly looked at that list. It was the first time I realized that out of those thirty people with whom we'd exchanged cards—people who were our world ten years before—twenty-eight of them were dead.

I hadn't thought of it in those terms. I hadn't sat down and said, "This is what's happening to my life." But I had been present at the death of six of them, and I helped three of them die. I mean, I assisted in their deaths. It was the first time it hit me, how big this AIDS epidemic was in my own life and how valuable those friendships were, cumulatively. When Scott died in 1990, only seven of our friends had died at that point. It was between '90 and '93 that so many of the others died. It took me a good couple of years just to get through that new grieving process of that huge loss.

What has been interesting has been to watch my father's reaction to all of this. He wrote me a letter after Scott died. My father is not the most expressive person that I've ever met. I have a lot of his characteristics! But in that letter he wrote to me that parents always like to be able to say to a child, "I know what you're going through," to have the experience to help a child go through it. Yet he said, "One of the things that bothers me most at this point is that I can't be that for you, because your mother's still alive. I don't know what it means to lose the person who means the most to you in the world." For my father to equate my relationship with Scott to his with my mother was a huge step for him. And for me, it was an opening of our relationship. Since that time, as a number of other friends whom my father knew have died, I have shared different stories with my father.

A few years ago, he said to me, "How do you do it? Why do you keep making friendships, knowing people are going to die?" And I said, "Why do you ask?" And he said, "Because I've never had that experience. A lot of people are starting to die who are my friends now, but I'm in my seventies and I'm learning to expect that. But I don't know how you, in your twenties and thirties and forties, can come to accept that."

My response surprised even me. I said, "I think by being able to share time and learn to love someone and then to be present with them as they deal with the kinds of issues that we as a society like to put over in the corner and pretend don't exist, to be present with them as they deal with their own mortality, and for them to be open to you to talk about what they're feeling, thinking, and experiencing, all of that is the most wonderful human experience you could possibly have. What it does is give you the doorway into the very core meaning of life."

When you're so busy living, you don't think about what life is all about. But when you're forced to stop and think about the end of life, you start understanding what it is that's so valuable. It's not having a nice dinner; it's the conversation that you have over the dinner. It's not going to a nice resort; it's being free to spend time, uncluttered by work and everything else, with another person so that you get to know them and so that their life stories become part of your life story and so that both of your life stories keep building on each other.

It has strengthened me. A lot of difficult things in the work world don't bother me. Hard relationships that we have with bureaucracies and other things—situations that, for example, bring an agency like Vermont CARES right to the brink—those situations don't bother me. I'm immune to what passes as stress for most people. What matters is what we're doing, what we do every day in our relationships with the people with whom we work or share our lives. What matters is that we're honest and we're direct and we know that what we're doing makes a difference, whether it's in our life or the life of someone else. All of this other stuff, it's just a lot of noise, that's all it is. Just a lot of noise. And that's one of the things I learned from Scott and from other friends who have dealt with the ends of their lives and have shared that with me.

In fact, I now have a much better understanding of how each of us impacts others, in ways that are as permanent as anything human can be. I will be here, as Scott will be here, forever. While we have no physical offspring, our interactions with people have had an impact on who they are, and they will have an impact on generation after generation after generation. That belief by some Native Americans that we are all part of one large spirit—I'm starting to believe that that's really true. We come into the world with some little wedge of that spirit, and our whole life is about shaping and growing and having many of those other little wedges of spirit impact us so that when we leave, we just go back into that larger and larger spirit. I am still working on how to best describe how I think about it, but that's my raw interpretation of it.

Being there at the end of Scott's life and at the end of other people's lives, I gained a sense of the freeing of the physical horror that is the illness that they're going through. Those last few breaths are just releases, an escape from the limitations that we physically are under. That simple statement, that I wouldn't have to buy the ticket, represented in Scott's way what I've come to understand and learn over the years. I don't buy him tickets any more, but he goes to everything!

Letha E. Mills, M.D.

Dr. Letha Mills was the beloved hematologist/oncologist of several patients whose family members I met in the course of collecting stories for this volume. Also an expert in palliative care, Letha was the kind of rare doctor who still made house calls, and whose patients and their families were comfortable calling her by her first name. True to her generous nature, Letha carved out a large block of time in her tightly scheduled workday to talk to me about her experiences with death and about the emotions doctors must take on and live with when losing a high percentage of their patients to cancer.

How we doctors approach death is primarily based on what we've seen. My perspective of death has changed with time. It's really a very interesting evolution that I haven't seen talked about much. When you're in medical school and you're in residency, it seems as if people are pretty realistic about what *can* be accomplished in terms of the medical care of the patient. Then when you graduate from your residency and become responsible for people and for making final decisions for them, you become much, much more conservative, as if you have to be the patient's advocate. You might see that they're dying, but until it's absolutely certain, you're kind of the one person who can't not give them the benefit of the doubt.

A lot of times what happens is that the situation creates a break between the other health-care providers—nurses, house staff, people in training—and the attending physician, who's actually responsible for the sick person. The doctor may know intuitively or instinctively that something might not work or that something else might be futile. But the doctor will be the last person to say that because he or she is the only person who can really make that decision. So, if a nurse says, "Continuing this person on a respirator doesn't make any sense," the nurse can verbalize that, but nothing's going to change. If the doctor says, "This doesn't make any sense," then it's over. Doctors make decisions to stop the respirator, to let the person die. That's a very, very big decision and not something that anybody takes lightly. A doctor's ability to make that decision and feel comfortable with it changes with time. When you're right out of fellowship, you think that you can cure leukemia. You think that if you do it your way, you're going to do it. And so you get very aggressive. And an older doctor will say, "Why are you doing that?" Because they've learned that you can only go so far.

The example that comes to my mind is about a young doctor who was fresh out of one of the more aggressive medical programs. He had a patient in her sixties with acute leukemia. During therapy, the patient ended up in the ICU six times during the course of a month with pulmonary edema. Her lungs would fill up with fluid from a heart-related problem. The doctor's view of leukemia, however, was that we don't get chemotherapy in fast enough, that the cancer cells or the leukemia cells regenerate because we don't treat people quickly enough. A patient might be in the hospital for four to six weeks. They go home and generally we give them two or three weeks to recuperate before we re-treat. And the doctor said, "That's the problem."

His idea was, "Well, we should get people right back in here and give them more therapy as quickly as possible, because we're allowing the leukemia to regrow in between these periods of time." So he brought this poor lady back in a week after she'd been in the hospital for four to six weeks, and we treated her again. And she went into the ICU *again*. And I said to him, "What are you doing? She's probably going to die of her heart disease within the next year. Don't you want to give her some quality time at home?" His answer was, "She can die of her heart disease, but she's not going to die of leukemia if I have anything to say about it."

That is a perfect example of what happens. A lot of times, what we don't do when somebody nears the end of life is admit it to ourselves, to the patient, to the family, quickly enough. But it's always a retrospective issue, too. Sometimes we don't know that death is coming. But always when we have interviewed family members after a patient has died, they say, "We wish we had known sooner. We wish we would have known that he or she was dying." We doctors may think we failed because we didn't tell a patient that she was dying, but it's not always clear to us, either, until that moment. It's really hard to say to somebody, "This person is dying," when the person may live for a month. You're afraid to say to somebody, "Your loved one is dying," when he or she might not be. The interesting thing about saying something like that to the patient is that most of the time, the patient actually knows, on some level, whether they're admitting it to themselves. They know it better than anybody.

I've evolved over time in how I feel about people dying. A lot of it has been painful. It has meant taking time out to read books, to become existential and spiritual and to figure out what I believe in order to understand how to be okay with this dying process. I have been learning to accept that death is the culmination of life and that everybody's going to die. But nothing in the way we were raised prepares us for that fact. So it's taken me a long time. I've sat on the porch of my house and tried to talk to my patients who have died, asking them, "Am I doing the right thing? I hope you're okay. Will you help somebody else who is dying? Will you?" Occasionally, I feel like there is some response. I am not prone to parapsychological phenomena like some people are. You read books in which people say, "I had this sense." But I look for these things.

After one of my patients died, I attended the burial, and the casket was being lowered into the ground. She was being buried in a corner of the cemetery with lots and lots of trees. As people were saying a prayer, the sun just came out through the trees and hit *me* in the face, full force. For that moment in time, I had the sense of warmth and the sense that she was telling me, "It's okay." Experiences like that have happened to me more than once. Obviously, I can evoke them myself, but when the sun comes through a window or when it spreads over me in some way, it feels like that same patient is again telling me, "It's okay. It's okay."

I had another patient, named Steve, whom I dearly adored. He was in his fifties, and was a wildlife biologist who specialized in birds. Six months after Steve died, a red-breasted grosbeak began living around my house, and I saw it I don't know how many times during that time. It never failed to make me think of Steve. People in medicine are trained to not pay attention to such things. The scientific model is deeply ingrained in medicine now. From my perspective, it has been taken too far. But it is hard to be in an academic medical center and to feel that way because you're always fighting the people who are most clear cut about, "No you didn't see that. No, that was just physiologic." In fact, there are palliative-care doctors with whom I have met and trained under who are just the same way. They will tell a patient's family, "Oh, that was a physiologic response. There's no way that they (the patient) can hear you. There's no way they know you're in the room. If they die when you're in the bathroom, don't worry about a thing because it just was meant to be. It could happen any minute and it has nothing to do with you. They don't know whether you're there or not."

A palliative-care specialist I know had spent quite a long time telling a patient's wife—and he was trying to alleviate her suffering—"Ah, don't worry about it if you're not in the room because physiologically he doesn't know you're there anyway." A belief like that is absolutely the opposite of what Hospice says. What the doctor was saying was shocking to me. In the academic, medical world, that specialist is considered the *crème de la crème*. But I said, "I do believe that the patient knows, somewhere deep inside, that the family member is there, whether or not the patient can ever say it." It's just my gut reaction. You can take palliative care to the model of science, but I think *all* of medicine has moved too far to the non-Hospice model. We've been polarized for much too long, it seems to me.

I remember a patient who was dying of leukemia who was in his thirties. He was dying in a hospital. It took him a week to die. His wife—they had no kids—was by his side the entire time. Other people kept saying, "What's taking him so long?" Those people were uncomfortable with the dying process. But the man actually held on until his wife was surrounded by a lot of people who could give her support. She knew all the nurses very well; he'd been in the hospital a lot in the previous year, and so it was a very comforting place for her to be, and he really did seem to hang on until she was ready, until it seemed to be okay for her. I remember there was a period of time when I had three patients die within a month of each other, and he was one of them. That was one of the most wrenching times of my life. That was when I had to sit down and think it out, what I believed. That was when I started reading Eastern traditions. I bought the *Tibetan Book of Living and Dying*. I was feeling like, Why don't we help people get through this better? Why isn't there more help for doctors in training to understand dying? There's so much data out there.

You will spend, as a physician, as much time dealing with people who are dying as you will with people with pneumonia. But if you actually look in the textbooks, there are no chapters in the textbooks of medicine on dying. There are big chapters on pneumonia and antibiotics and everything else. But there isn't anything about, How does a person die? Palliative-care textbooks address the topic. But if you look at general medical books, for years they haven't even referred to people dying. They don't refer to the terminal phase of any illness, as if there was no terminal phase. So we all perpetuate the issue of not being comfortable that it is an okay time, ever, to say, "Yes, this is happening." It's why many of us have trouble with that. Part of the difficulty is not being able to afford to go through those emotions. Doctors can be kind of intimately involved, to a point, but then we have to carry out the rest of our day's activities. It's only when we actually hear that X person has died that we can't get away from the emotion of it. Doctors don't process the emotions like a family member does, who has been there a lot, up until that moment in time.

A patient died this weekend who was my age, and whom I'd known for the last six or seven years. She died of breast cancer at her home, and I was over there almost every day for the last five or six days. Her husband called me Sunday morning to tell me that she had died that morning. I burst into tears and he kept saying, "I'm so sorry. I'm really so sorry." He was perfectly calm and perfectly okay.

And I said, "You're not supposed to be saying this." And he said, "I'm sorry you have to go through this." He had been there day in and day out, and I think to him it was a blessing at that point that she had let go of her suffering and that he didn't have to anticipate dealing with any more of her physical suffering. So the husband was relieved, but the reality had just finally hit me.

I think the most difficult part of being around somebody who's dying is that you're afraid that you're going to get into a situation where they're going to be uncomfortable and you're not going to know what to do. Medicine and the environment of medicine are notoriously terrible for helping people deal with the death of patients. Another patient—also with leukemia—was a young man, fortyish, who was in one room on the hospital floor for three months. Every single day, he was there. He was a very detail-oriented person. He would give us a list every morning that showed us that he had just spent hours trying to put together things that probably had no bearing on one another. He would ask us if eating processed cereal had led to his leukemia or if it was because he was so busy that he didn't get enough exercise in the year before he was diagnosed. Things like that. He would sit there and try to come up with a physiologic reason about his illness. He was seeking answers and reasons.

It was an intense experience, because when we went through second- and third-line chemotherapy and it wasn't working, the patient's brother came in at the eleventh hour and started doing Internet searches and saying, "No, no, you can't give up." Yet at that point, the patient was actually ready to let go. He had had enough. He realized that we had been through all the experimental options and that yes, he could go to Sloan-Kettering if he wanted, or try something else, but that there really was nothing that was going to offer him a good shot at curing the disease. The patient was okay, but his brother was not.

The man died about a week later. I came in the next morning, and he was gone, his room was clean, and nobody—the house staff, the intern, the resident, or the nurses—said anything. Everybody was willing to sweep it under the carpet and not acknowledge it because that was the easiest thing to do. Each medical person has to deal with death in his or her own way, but none of us can avoid being impacted by a death like that. Yet there isn't any forum in which medical personnel are able to say, "How do you feel about the fact that Mr. So and So just died?"

Medicine has so many rewarding moments, but when somebody is dying in our health care system, there are not a lot of rewards on anybody's side. We actually have the Institute for Health Care Improvement that has decided to improve end-of-life care as a project, and our hospital bought into it. It's a year-long project. You actually pay money to participate in it. It's a quality-improvement method that says "This is research. Try something that you think might work. Try it, pilot it for a short period of time. Assess it. Decide that it did or didn't do something, and then move on," instead of the approach, "We're going to do a big research study and do fifteen implementations and analyses and whatnot."

Forty-three hospitals were in this project. Some were Hospice hospitals. Some were private hospitals. Some were academic centers. There was a team at each site, and we would decide what we wanted to study, what we thought we could improve, and then we would have some measures for outcome. They wanted very specific numbers, such as decreasing the experience of pain in a patient by 50 percent. That means you have to have some baseline data saying how many patients have pain. Then you try something and then you reassess it to see whether people still have pain at the same percentage. We got into this process, and as part of it, we decided to go back and ask people who'd had a family member die between six and twelve months ago in our hospital to come and do a focus group so that we could learn what their experiences had been. We hoped to figure out what areas we as a system needed to improve on instead of saying just, "Well, maybe this is or isn't a problem."

So we brought family members back, and two or three of them brought up the fact that the medical person who came into the room and actually did the pronouncing of the death was an intern who usually would say, "Yes, there is no heartbeat. Yes, there is no—" It was such a cold approach that it had really bothered the family members. He came in, just said, "Yup." He didn't make eye contact. Then he walked out again. Obviously he was terribly uncomfortable.

Family members talked about how much it had colored the experience of that moment in time. So we developed a pronouncement card that we laminated and gave to all the new interns. We want interns to recognize, before they go into the room, what an incredible moment this is for the family members and to try to somehow acknowledge their experience. Even if it's only a hand touch on the shoulder and an "I'm sorry"—anything to make it a more human experience.

It is remarkable that we don't teach that. In every other way in medicine, we teach like that. We start an IV, and we follow the approach of "See one, do one, teach one." If you need an IV then we say, "Here, watch how I do it." But no one ever says, "Gee, how do you go in and pronounce somebody dead, and what do you say to the family member and how do you feel and how do you process it and what do you do?" These are incredible human emotions that just totally go by in medical school. So we brought this up and presented it at one of our conferences. It was really very interesting because we presented the family focus group data, and doctors started to raise their hands and say, "I remember my first experience." We had a really good discourse.

Medical people clearly want to talk about issues surrounding death, but no one ever gives them the opportunity to do it. It's not just patients and their families who need to. It's doctors who want to talk about it, too, in some acceptable forum. It is just as difficult an experience from our perspective.

When I was doing palliative-care training in a center that had a big palliative-care program, I was working with two residents in family practice who were with me. We talked about a patient who had just been admitted. I told them that I would ask the patient what he thought about life after death. The residents would look at me and say, "You did? You asked them that?" And I'd say, "Well, yeah. I don't have trouble at this point in time asking people what they believe or what they think happens."

One of the Hospice chaplains said that patients don't seem to want to talk, to any great degree, about what's going to happen to them after they die. I thought, People don't want to talk to the Hospice chaplain? Wow. I would have thought that topic would have come up with virtually every person. That patient's asking, "What is the meaning of my life?" is kind of part and parcel to "What's going to happen to me when I die? What does this all mean?" The chaplain said that most of the time patients are more concerned with "Am I going to be in pain?" or with relationships that are ending or are about to end and with how other people are going to cope.

I have spent a lot of time trying to figure out, Is there life after death? Obviously I don't know. But I believe it's the only thing that makes sense. Otherwise, there is no justice and there is no understanding in this world. People suffer and people die. People are impoverished and die of starvation all over the world. But it doesn't make any sense unless it's a process and they'll come back in a different way and a different sense, unless we're all on some sort of spiritual journey of our soul toward some higher plane and we go through lives to figure out what that next step is, what we need to learn from this life.

I had a patient who was in her twenties who died of a really horrible sarcoma. She had had a very difficult life. She'd been sexually abused by her brothers when she was little. She was beautiful, with long, blond hair. She had been diagnosed with a sarcoma and was treated in Boston and the Boston people said to her, "You need a bone-marrow transplant." I first met her when she came to my hospital. She did have a transplant. But ultimately she relapsed.

She had been living with a guy who left her when he realized she was not going to live. And then she formed another relationship with a truck driver who did stay by her until she died. But she went in and out of abusing medications and alcohol, and that behavior came out in the period of time before the disease came back but after she had had all the therapy. She was trying to cope, but she ended up on the psychiatric in-patient unit.

She and I started to have conversations about "Do you believe?" I gave her a book by psychiatrist Brian Weiss. It's really an interesting book. It's about reincarnation. It's a story about a woman for whom he did hypnotherapy because she had allergies to virtually every medication known to man. He thought he was doing regression to a time in which she was abused as a child. It turned out that he had said to her at one point, "Go back to when this started," and she started going through past lives. It took him about ten years to write the book, to actually come out. He was a psychiatrist who lived in Florida. He was actually very into neurobiology, brain chemistry and that kind of thing. So for him to come out and tell this story was a big deal. But she knew things and would say things during these sessions with Weiss that nobody could have known.

Weiss had had a child who had died at twenty-one days of life from a congenital heart defect. The woman, in her trance, would tell him things like "You had a child who died." He had no pictures, no anything, and nobody who worked around him knew anything about it. Every time she remembered a past life and how she had died, she lost one of her phobias. So this got Weiss into this treatment as sort of a therapy. And because the mind is a funny thing, you can get people to let go of things in many ways, using his approach. Weiss's book had started me thinking, so I gave it to this girl. She read it and felt so much better about everything that she had been through in her life. She said to me, "You know, I'll bet you were my mother in a past life." And I thought, You know, I'll bet you're right.

I have to say that to this day, I think what brings me the most comfort when people are dying—especially young people, when they're dying—is that this is all part of a bigger process. I have a really hard time believing that death is the final experience that happens to a person.

What Brian Weiss said after he wrote the first book was that lots of people have come up to him and told him their stories, and that they really are mystical, truly mystical stories. In one story, a dying young man began talking rather incoherently to his friend, Michael. He hadn't seen Michael in years. They used to play together in the summers. Michael lived across the country. It turned out after this young man died that Michael had died something like forty-eight hours earlier, on the other side of the country. There are all sorts of stories like that, such as about people who have woken up and suddenly known that someone must have died, even though that person wasn't expected to die. They are incredible stories, and lots and lots of these stories exist.

I started listening to tapes the Fetzer Institute had sent to me.

The one on human consciousness was fascinating. It talked about how our Western society and our scientific minds have tried to make everything into a time-space continuum so that we can box up the mind and the emotions and can define them based on physiology and how all the synapses work. The tape included an interview with a neurophysiologist who talked about the fact that people who are physiologically dead in an ICU—in a near-death experience—can later describe who was in the room at the time and all sort of other things, and yet they had had no brain activity at the time they were unconscious. Doctors have actually hooked electrodes up to the person and have proven that there is no brain activity during that period of time that the patient later can define.

So Fetzer staff people were doing studies in which they would scientifically prove this phenomenon. They would put things in people's rooms and interview them later on to find out whether they saw that in the room, to prove that there was something there. A Hospice director, a doctor, in New Hampshire had a near-death experience when her second child was being born. The doctor has given an amazing talk about it to many people. I have heard her talk, and it's an incredibly moving story about what she went through.

I've read about a few monks in Tibet who are so good at meditation that one of them appeared dead for a week before his body began to actually act like it was dead. People around him couldn't find a heartbeat on him, and he wasn't breathing. But for a long time, he didn't go through any sort of rigor mortis or any distortion of his body. He had been able to actually meditate while he was sleeping, and he had an incredible control over his sleep-wake state. Medical personnel actually flew over to Tibet with all of their equipment to try to figure out whether there was any discernable electrical activity anywhere in the body, using our Western technology. This story sort of slowly filtered out. But the monk had actually begun to clearly die, by that point. But for those seven days, he wasn't dying, but he wasn't breathing, and he didn't seem to have a heartbeat. It potentially redefines what your mind can do to your body. I think we don't explore that area enough. It's one of our biggest problems, actually, in this medical autonomy. We only say,

"You need to know everything there is to know about the side effects of these drugs."

My mother is one of those people to whom you say that a drug has a potential side effect, and she'll get it. Sure enough, she took Cytoxan and Prednisone for her lymphoma when she was in the hospital. She never had one whit of nausea until the pharmacist said, "Cytoxan can cause nausea." She said, "It can?" Then she began to throw up uncontrollably, and she couldn't take another dose.

One patient of mine who was forty-six died this weekend. She was incredibly frustrated and upset by not being able to carry on activities of daily living. Her youngest daughter, who was in second grade, had dropped a paper on the floor. The woman said it took everything she had to bend over and pick up that paper, and she felt useless. I said to her, "Wait a minute here. We are not defined by what we can physically carry out, despite what the world would say. Whether you can cook or whether you can't, you're still the same person, and you're still loved by people." We get so defined by our roles and what we can carry out that when we can't carry them out, we feel like we should die.

I tried to reassure her that people just wanted her to be here and that it was okay if she couldn't do something at this moment in her life. If you have a newborn baby, you still love it even though it can't do a thing. The baby has never done anything. And it's not just the belief that the baby is going to turn into something that you can love more that makes you love it. If you truly love someone, you can get frustrated but you don't love them less because they can't pick up a paper anymore.

I've had two especially extraordinary deaths in my experience as a doctor. One was a woman who went through treatment while also trying to understand what was going on. She read books up the wazoo. She would go through the Rachel Naomi Ramen book, *Kitchen Table Wisdom*. She actually gave me the book. It's a wonderful book. Rachel Naomi Ramen is my role model. My patient read that book and lots and lots of other books. She would come see me with anxieties about her medical condition, and yet throughout, she was trying to process the concept of dying through writing, reading, and painting. She used her creativity to deal with what she felt. She sought guidance from others to help her accept her own death, but the funny thing is, she didn't need to do that. She thought she did, but she had already gotten to that place of understanding on her own.

She worked hard to get to where she was. She actively decided to not have any more therapy. It was hard work for her all the way along, but most people don't go through that amount of work. By the time she decided that she had had enough, she was really okay with it. It was just the most incredible experience for me. She radiated love that said, "I'm okay with this." She took the burden away from the rest of us who might otherwise have felt guilty that she still had the disease. She had all these things wrong with her body, but she was okay. "I'm okay," she would say, "I love you. I love you all." It was as if she were saying, "Let's celebrate what we have together, not what we're losing." Although she would cry, too. But all of it was honest emotions.

I think a lot of people, at whatever stage or age they've reached, have unfinished issues that they haven't dealt with that somehow impact their ability to feel peace at the time of death. Some people may not even be able to see what it is that bothers them. But you're not going to change people like that at the eleventh hour and get them to be insightful and introspective.

The other person I knew who had an incredible death was a man in his forties who had acute leukemia. He had three young daughters. But from the time he was diagnosed, he had a very positive attitude, very upbeat. When it was time to mow the lawn, he would trim the perimeter first so that it would be easier to mow if somebody else had to do the rest. When it was sugaring time in March, he, who had always done all the sugaring, taught his daughter how to do it. There was some subliminal discussion, but not a lot of overt "In case I'm not here, you ought to know how to do this." Sometimes I think he had more overt discussions with his wife: "You ought to know about this." It wasn't like he was preparing to die. But he was. For two years, he was being really responsible and figuring it out. Most of the time he was well, or recovering from chemotherapy, so he was emotionally okay, if not physically so.

Then it came to a point where he relapsed after a bone-marrow transplant. He went through a very severe depression when he relapsed. It was as if all his upbeat behavior and his "I'm going to beat this. I'm going to beat this" had all totally failed him, and he had no coping mechanisms for three months. He was really very dependent and very whiny, all of those things we hate to see. But then he sort of climbed out of that and became his old self again but made sure that all of these things were done for his family. When he got to a point where he was spending a lot of time in the hospital, either because of fevers or needing blood or whatever, he said, "Okay, I'm not going to go this next step. I have no quality of life left."

He died in the hospital, but everybody knew that this was happening because he said, "Okay, I'm ready now to stop transfusions." For the next forty-eight hours, people paraded through his room. Hundreds of people came to see him, and he would wake up and smile at them and recognize them. He was able to say good-bye to all sorts of people in a very open way. He had something special to say to each person and was not afraid to say it. He hugged them. But when he went into his dying process, where he could barely wake up, he would still wake up, connect with your eyes, and then give you this sweet smile and close his eyes again. It was like up until the end he was thinking as much of other people as he could. I guess what we think of as a good death, at least for both of those two people, is when they help put us at ease with their process of dying. What I consider a good death is that I feel okay that this is happening, and that I can accept it because the dying person is okay with it.

My father died in 1983, when I was a fellow. I was the doctor in the family. He was a doctor, too. I went home with all of these thoughts of "Gee, you have to open up. And you have to accept that you're dying and you have to go through all of these things." I tried to get him to open up even a little bit, but he was not going to admit it. He would just look at me and say, "So what are we going to do now? How am I going to get stronger?" I'd say, "Well, we could get a physical therapist to come in." "Great idea! Great. Let's do that." Then somewhere along the line, I realized that I just had to let it go. He did not think that dying was okay because that meant leaving us was okay, and it wasn't okay that he was leaving us and so he was not going to say, "This is okay." He was seventy years old. We were all grown. All those things were in place, but it was not okay. And he lived his whole life with this "I'm a strong man" belief. It wasn't like he was capable of opening up and saying, "I'm scared."

I've come to recognize that you can only expect so much change in somebody who is dying, in terms of what he or she is willing to talk about or accept. What I try to do now is have some sort of a what-if conversation so that I know how that individual feels but still try to support where the person is at that moment in time—"Yes, we will work on getting you down to have a bone-marrow transplant or do this experimental protocol"—to not rip the rug out from under them and say, "No, that's crazy," but to gently kind of say, "Yes, we will work toward that but what do you feel about X, Y, or Z if this should happen or if we should not be able to do that?" I try to get a sense about where they're at without taking their hope away.

Unfortunately, it seems like we need an incredible revamping of medicine. What's happening now is a step in the right direction, with the work that's being done to teach doctors to communicate. It's amazing how many people will tell you, "I went to the doctor, and he didn't seem to be listening to what I had to say," or they'll tell you that a doctor latched onto one statement that they mentioned and didn't hear anything else.

We can do things to help doctors learn to communicate. Some of that is being done. How we get doctors to value the whole person is in part changing the way that we test people. We doctors are so factually oriented. One of the saddest things I watched was when a doctor I respected stopped running an oncology course he had taught for years. He said, "I got tired of students saying I was too touchy-feely." He had done things like bringing a cancer patient in and having the students interview the patient. Basically, the students would say, "We don't want to interview somebody. We want to know what facts we need to know about breast cancer. What are you going to test us on?"

As long as assessment or testing systems or our criteria for how well patients are doing are so factually oriented, then that's the material on which doctors are going to continue to rely. Medicine is turning into evidence-based medicine, outcomes. Medical people are big into outcomes. A doctor says, "You have prostate cancer. Do you want to have surgery?" Then the doctor walks the patient through the percentage odds for each step, to help patients make a decision. Instead, doctors need to say, "Wait a minute. You're not a thousand people. You're one individual." So I don't believe it when I hear, "Well, if you get treated for your prostate cancer, you can add eight months of time to your life." That's only a statistical response.

I heard Larry Dossey and Rachel Naomi Ramen speak at a conference once. Rachel Naomi Ramen talked about facilitating healing. She said that Western medicine has become exceptionally good at treating illnesses and diagnosing technology, but that we need to recognize that we're not here to *fix* people. We're here to facilitate healing. We doctors also need to know that it's okay to bring where we are and who we are to a patient encounter. We don't have to be this person in a white coat who sits there and knows everything and doesn't get involved. It's okay to bring ourselves to that encounter. The only way that we're not going to burn out in medicine is to work with someone, to facilitate their healing, to not say, "You have something that is broken. It's my job to fix it, and if I don't fix it, then I've failed," which is the corollary for why doctors get burned out.

A lot of the way I have changed by accompanying people through death is that I try to realize that I have got to live for today because I don't know what's going to happen tomorrow. We all ought to be aware that life is tenuous. Just because you take care of your body does not mean anything. Running X number of miles per day, eating low fat, doing all these things—there seems to be this concept in our society that if you take care of yourself, you'll live forever, and that's not true. I see it day in and day out. There's no correlation on a case-by-case basis. You can make big statistical correlations, but there are many people who have done a wonderful job taking care of their bodies who have died prematurely. So try to live day to day.

I struggle with trying to take care of myself, realizing that I can't take care of other people well unless I take care of myself, but again, I struggle against a system that doesn't want me to take care of myself. It only wants me to take care of other people. But I am realizing how important that self-care is. It's the most difficult part of my life—trying to figure out how to do it. I am drained at the end of several days in a row, chronically. You see new patients with newly diagnosed breast cancer. It's an intense emotional experience, and they're asking a lot of questions. Some of it is just airing things over and over—what they might lose—and decision making. A lot of highly intelligent people think, I should be able to change X, Y, and Z thing and be okay, so just tell me what it is and I'll do it. You hear them and walk them through the choices. But part of me is realizing that the choices probably are not going to do it. What you've got to do is try to do what you want to do each day and interact with the people that you want to interact with and try to let everything else go. Because in the end, no matter what you do, there's an ending. It's true.

Sometimes we have what appears to be a home run and the disease is at bay. But then the person will turn around and become an alcoholic because he has so many other issues with which he is now struggling. I believe we ought to start people—regardless of whether they are potentially curable or not—with the same tenets and the same support systems. What are your goals for therapy? What do you believe in? What are your support systems? How do we enhance that? And what information do you need to live a fuller life? And if you get cured of your disease, along this path—*wonderful!* We all can only gain. It's a win-win situation, if you can get to know who you are, what you believe in, what meaning you have in your life. Then if I cure you of this disease or if your disease gets cured by whatever you do, wonderful. But you still have got—at some point down the line—to address these questions.

Why not do this when you first meet people? Why does palliative care, by definition, have to be for someone who is incurable? We're spending too much time, as a society, focusing on various drug therapies and not on how people deal with their bodies, their souls, their meaning in life. We have a lot of work to do.

Anita F. Bonna

Anita Bonna, an R.N., was recommended to me by a person who knew her and who felt that Anita's story of the death of her husband, Cliff, should be included in my book. After decades of living with Hodgkin's disease, Cliff had died of a rapidly moving non-Hodgkin's lymphoma. As with all the other people I interviewed for this book, when I contacted her, Anita graciously agreed to share with me the painful but tender details of the drama and decisions that defined Cliff's final hours. She invited me to her house, fed me tea, and told me her story so that others might learn from it and be better able to make their own decisions if they ever found themselves in a similar situation.

I married Cliff after he was diagnosed with Hodgkin's disease. We found out that he had cancer while we were dating. We dated for five years before we got married, and we got married in between radiation treatments. They do the upper body and they take a break and then they do the lower body, so we got married during that time. It was 1975. So Cliff had Hodgkin's disease for our entire marriage and even a little bit before that. We had known each other for a total of twenty-three years when he died.

At some point during our marriage, the side effects of his radiation started to show up, causing a vascular necrosis of both of Cliff's hips, which means that the circulation to that particular area is diminished. Cliff had a number of hip surgeries—I think a total of five in all, over the years. He was a skier, so that condition changed his life. We took annual jaunts to Boston for hip surgery. And then he had a recurrence. Another lymph node showed up malignant, positive for Hodgkin's disease. So that was removed. Then another lymph node showed up as malignant quite a few years after he had finished all the treatment. Doctors took that out. It, too, was positive for Hodgkin's disease. I think they treated that area with some local radiation. And then things were okay again. There was a stable period of time and, of course, life went on. You know, you're thinking about buying a house, thinking about children, working, and so forth. I was working as a nurse. But then damage similar to what had occurred to Cliff's hips showed up in his heart, in his chest.

Doctors tried to treat him medically. He was a young man. He was one of the strongest men, in a quiet way, that I've ever known. I've often thought that Cliff was well beyond his years in age. If there are old souls walking this planet, I think he was one of them. His whole adult life was spent dealing with all of this. Cliff was maybe twenty when he was first diagnosed, early twenties. And he died when he was forty-three. But Cliff had an incredible spirit. He was a very solid man with a tremendous will to live. I tend to complain. I tend to be—had been, at least in my past—negative. Cliff loved life, no matter what it dished out to him.

No physician had ever, over all those years, said his cancer was terminal. We didn't even know the cancer was back. They didn't either, until they got him in for that last final open-heart surgery. That's when he was diagnosed. The final diagnosis, and the reason Cliff died, was a non-Hodgkin's lymphoma, which I understand is potentially a fatal, rapid, very aggressive type, very different from Hodgkin's disease. He was diagnosed nine months prior to his death. He went through the final round of very aggressive chemotherapy of about six or seven months. Everybody was hopeful. I remember medical personnel saying, "If you get through the first year after we finish, that will be a good sign." But we didn't get that far. It was less than two months—maybe a month and a half—after he finished treatment that he had emergency surgery for a bowel obstruction, and that's when they opened him up and basically closed him up and said the cancer was everywhere.

When I say the cancer was everywhere, it was. And there were complications from the surgery. He wound up in an ICU in critical condition, in crisis, and they said, "You know, he's not doing well, and his life is going to end." That was the first he'd heard of it and the first I'd heard of it.

The shift in perspectives started the minute they got him into the ICU, where I got the feeling that there was pressure on Cliff to die. They had made a decision that this was the end of the road. Cliff was not in that mind-set. I was not in that mind-set, either. Cliff needed more time. It was happening too quickly. The powers that be had decided that everything that was going to be done for him had now been done. I had a very ill husband, but a conscious one who was saying, "I am not ready to die." Cliff had a Living Will, but the doctors never asked about it. They knew what a fighter Cliff was. A member of the ICU medical team said to me at one point, "That's why Cliff's in this unit in the first place, because we know what a fighter he is. And we know that's what he wanted. But now the time has come for this to be over."

To this day I don't understand that conclusion. I have no idea how we couldn't come up with a compromise for Cliff. It was a desperate time. And it was never even that Cliff wanted to die at home. Cliff didn't think he was dying. The doctors made it sound like they were honoring this dying man's last wish to die in his own bed. I know that they knew that wasn't the case. This was a power struggle. I think there are probably many, many situations that occur like this in hospitals. The difference, I think, is that most patients are not conscious when it gets to this point, so the medical team approaches family members to make those decisions. But Cliff was still awake, still making decisions and interacting and giving feedback. He was motioning. He was medicated, and they tried to bring that up, as if he were incompetent. Cliff was as competent as I've ever known him to be. Cliff was pointing for the board to write on. Cliff was making it very clear: "I am not ready. Do whatever you have to do, but I don't want to die today."

At the last medical meeting—and I can't remember how many we had; this was the final one after many—all of Cliff's physicians were there. Somebody from risk management was there. The social workers were there. The oxygen person. Who wasn't there? I don't know.

I was exhausted by this point, and frightened. It was unbelievable. But my sister, my nephew, and a colleague of mine were with me. I had been severely reprimanded by the surgeon, who asked how dare I prolong this man's life like this. He was so angry with me—yelling at me the night before on the telephone—that I wasn't even able to tell him, "This isn't my decision. This is Cliff's." I never got a chance to say it in this meeting, either.

They called me into the final meeting to tell me that his condition had deteriorated to the point—and it had gotten worse overnight— where now what they were going to do was administer this paralyzing drug and that medical protocol allowed them to do that. They knew Cliff would never wake up again and that he would be dead by that afternoon. They said I should go in and say good-bye to my husband while he was still awake. And I said, "I can't give you permission to do that. Cliff isn't ready for that. He has told me. He is not ready to die."

I tried to talk about options. I mean, I went through everything. "If it's the insurance money, I will pay out of pocket. Put the paper in front of me. Take him off Blue Cross. If it's the fact that you've got a terminal man in the ICU, put him in a room on one of the floors. Take him out of here. Do whatever is necessary." No. There was no other option. They were giving the drug. They had already stopped some medicines. I don't know where they got the permission to do that, but they had already stopped some treatment, and they wanted me to go in and say good-bye to him. I refused. I had just spoken with Cliff. I said to him, "Cliff, push has come to shove. This is what they want to do." Cliff made it clear, "Don't do this." So I said they couldn't do it. They tried to talk me into it. And they basically said to me, "You don't know what you're going to go through or how difficult this is going to be for you if you sign him out of this hospital." They would not say, "No, we will not give the medicine, the paralyzing drug." So I couldn't leave him there. I hired an ambulance and told Cliff what I was doing. He agreed, and we took him out of the hospital. The hospital made me sign. I probably signed everything away. I have no idea what I signed. But I signed.

They were convinced that Cliff wouldn't survive the twenty-minute ambulance ride home. They were positive he would die in the ambulance. They only gave him like a 500 cc bag of solution. It was half empty. They made no follow-up plans. They didn't ever want to see him again. I had nothing. No oxygen. No meds. No nothing.

It's very vague in my mind how many people were involved. I rode in the ambulance with Cliff and his sister and two other people, I think. Two people from the hospital came with us because I had borrowed a hospital ventilator. I had their equipment. When we got Cliff to the house, a lot of people had already arrived. Some of them were colleagues and family members. I don't have a clue who was there. A lot of people were around, and they got Cliff into his bed. From there we had thirteen hours. It was November 12. Cliff died at 3:10 the next morning.

I have lots of photos of that night. We had a tape recorder going, and music was being played. Cliff's best friend, Peter, was there. They had grown up together. When they were young boys, they each got their first guitar. Growing up, they had played music together. Cliff didn't play that night, not the night he was dying.

The phone had been ringing, and people had been calling. Word had gotten out that Cliff was dying, that he was coming home and that we were in this acute-crisis situation. I can remember taking that call and saying to Peter, "I don't know if you'll make it." But he said, "I'm going to try."

Peter played a number of the old songs from when Cliff and I first met. One of them was *our* song, "My Creole Belle." Cliff lifted his hands. He was awake but on morphine, so he was probably in a very funny state of mind. But Cliff was playing a guitar, even though there was no guitar in his hands. And Cliff was mouthing the words to the song. He put his arm around me and hugged me. I have pictures of that embrace. He put his arm around me, and he held me with a strength that was unbelievable—so tight, it almost hurt. And he kissed me. You wouldn't think, to look at him, that he had that strength left. Oh, he did. He did.

We had all that Friday late afternoon, Friday evening, Friday night. And he acknowledged everybody. I mean, when my sister was in the room, he tried to reach for things that she had given him. It was clear that he knew she was there. Oh, he was alert. When Gary, our neighbor, a pharmacist, came by with some medication, he shook Cliff's hand and he said, "He's so strong."

At one point, somebody said, "Shall we pray?" So everybody in the room joined hands and prayed. I think we started with the "Our Father," and then somebody said the Twenty-third Psalm, which was one of Cliff's favorites. We were both Catholic. Cliff had been an altar boy, and I had gone to Catholic school for twelve years. It was funny because nobody seemed to remember how to start the Twenty-third Psalm. And then somebody finally did. So we had, at one time, a whole room full of people all holding hands with Cliff in the bed. I was in the bed, too, as was the dog. Other people were seated on the bed, all praying.

It had been a grueling two or three days. People went to sleep on the floor in sleeping bags and on blankets and pillows. The house was full of people. Finally the bedroom was empty, except for Cliff and me. The ventilator was pumping. He was dozing and kind of falling in and out of sleep. I decided at one point to turn the light off. I was beginning to feel like I could close my eyes and go to sleep beside him. I turned the light off, but I never did fall asleep. Very shortly thereafter, I heard a very funny sound, like gushing wind. It was a sound that I had not heard before. I turned the light back on and saw that Cliff was motioning in the air, trying to pull the air with both of his hands toward his face. I woke up the nurses sleeping in the living room. It must have been around 2:00 A.M.

The tube had developed a leak. I asked about getting Cliff back to the hospital. We called the ambulance to take him back, but one of the nurses said that by that point, Cliff had been oxygen deprived for so long that he would never live; the transport from the bed onto a stretcher would have killed him. She was clear about that.

The nurse stayed with me. Two other R.N.s were there with us, too. There were six of us in the room. Cliff was conscious for that last hour—in and out, but conscious enough that when the tube came out, he sat right up in the bed and woke up bright. His eyes were open, and he said, "Help me, help me, help me." I didn't even know he could speak. He said, "Help me, help me, help me. I need a new tube." And that's when he died.

I remember the horror in every detail. Other people forgot the specifics over time. The sad facts of it were sort of lost to them. What they remembered was the beauty of that last thirteen hours. From right after Cliff's death until even a year or two later, people who were present during that last thirteen hours would still cry, remembering the beauty of those hours. One of them said later, "I have never experienced anything like that. I have never been moved like that." What was going on in that room, the feeling in that room that night, was enough to bring people who were part of that to tears months, a year, two years later. They had forgotten the excruciating details.

After Cliff died, I stayed with him. His death was so sudden. Not only was he not ready, I wasn't ready. I needed my time with Cliff to make my own good-byes. So after he died, I just went to sleep beside him, in our bed, and almost two days went by.

The other people who were here were beside themselves that I was doing that. I didn't intentionally upset them. I remember them trying to come in to talk with me. I remember saying to my colleague and friend, "What are you doing here? Go home. Your work here is done. You have a family at home. You have children. There's nothing more you can do. I need to sleep with Cliff. We need to get our rest."

People kept coming in and trying to talk to me. I didn't really grasp everything that was going on. To me it was the most natural time; it was the most natural thing to do. It was less than two days that I slept there with Cliff. But it was a fairly long time. I had no concept of the time at that point. I remember opening the window. It was cold; it was November. They wanted to take Cliff away. They would have had had to take my life first.

I wasn't conscious of the amount of time passing as I lay there. I just knew it was my healing time with Cliff. I remember very distinctly that his legs and arms got cold fairly quickly. But Cliff's chest was still warm. Now, I don't know what the mind does under shock. I don't know. I don't pretend to be an expert in that area, but I can remember saying to them, "You're not taking Cliff until the warmth is gone out of his chest and every other part is cold."

I had to go out to the living room at one point, and I had to be very strong and stand my ground. Two or three people were there. One of them was Cliff's sister. They were talking about the health department. I tried to be sensitive. I think the others had gone. I remember coming out and saying to Cliff's sister, "I don't mean to be insensitive. I know he's your brother. I know you love him. I know this is difficult, but this is *my* house and he's *my* husband and this is the way it has to be. I am not ready for him to go and he's not ready to go."

I asked them to please just not keep coming in and bothering me. They wanted to take him; they were trying to talk me into letting him go. I don't remember much of it. Very little. I do remember calling a friend of mine whose daughter was in mortuary school. I had the presence of mind, even with all of that, because I knew they were pressuring me. I called her and she gave me some guidelines. She said, "Open the window." And I said, "Can they make him go? Is there any health department regulation?" She said, "No. I don't think there is. I think you're all right." So I opened the window.

Finally, when that warmth was gone from his chest, when he was ready, I was completely at peace, and ready for them to take him.

I called the funeral home Monday morning, and by the time they got here it was around 1:00. A physician had come to pronounce Cliff dead. The funeral people came out to the house, and they were very nice. They said, "Nita, do you want anything?" I told them that I wanted the nightshirt that he had on and the blanket in which he had been wrapped. I asked them to take those things off and leave them with me. And they said, "Anita, the blanket is soiled." I said, "I don't care." They left me one of the blankets and said they were going to take the other one because it was so soiled. I said that was fine. They said, "Do you want us to cover his head or not?" And I said, "No, don't cover his head. Just cover him to his chest." Then they took him away. It was perfect; it was time for him to go. I felt that at that point his spirit was ready.

Cliff's presence was in the house for a long time, even after they took his body. I would come home from work and find it so comforting being there. I felt Cliff in the house very strongly for a long, long time. I had a dream. I think it was a dream. I don't know what it was, but I will call it a dream because I think that's what everybody else would call it. Whatever it was, I was in bed and I woke up and got out of bed and I went out to the living room. I can remember getting out of bed and putting my slippers on. I remember the walk from the bedroom. I remember exactly where I stood. And I could see Cliff in the kitchen.

It was daytime in the kitchen. It was actually nighttime, and I was in bed. But it was daytime in the kitchen in that dream or vision or whatever it was. Cliff was in the kitchen doing the dishes, standing right there, in the same clothes. I stood right in the little foyer that goes into the bathroom and I said, "Cliff, you know what? They're trying to tell me that you're gone. They're all trying to tell me that you're gone, and I knew you weren't gone." And then I went back to bed.

I saw Cliff other times, like that. Another time in a dream, I was at my sister's house. Again, I watched myself get out of bed and go to my sister's window. She has blinds on her windows, unlike me; I have curtains. The blind was closed tight. I stood by the window and Cliff was behind me. He came behind me. I never saw him. He came up behind me. And I cracked the blind, a little bit, and it was brilliant sunshine behind the blind. The whole room was dark. So black. I didn't want to open the blind, but Cliff helped me. He stood behind me. He didn't speak to me. We never exchanged words. But when that blind was cracked, when you would look out of it, there was brilliant sunshine outside.

I'm guessing, but I'd say that dream occurred three months after Cliff's death. By then, I was managing. I was working. I was functioning. Oh, I've had other times with him. I can remember seeing him driving home from Boston. I remember seeing Cliff, in the sky, just kind of elevated over the highway. Maybe it was my mind, I don't know. But I remember that Cliff had his suede brown jacket on. He had different clothes on each of those times.

Another time, he was dressed in white. And he was in his old white car. I was at a meeting and I was parking the car. It was my garden-society meeting. And I was just pulling into the parking space. I was in the town of Quechee. You know, it sort of didn't matter where it was. I don't know what people make of these kinds of things. Everybody can make what they will of them. I just know how Cliff appeared to me. I know what a tremendous help his presence was to me, in a way you couldn't really put into words.

Cliff's complex death, and the fact that Cliff never accepted his death, compounded and prolonged my grief. When he was going through the last chemotherapy, I would say, "I'm afraid you're dying." And he would say to me, "Nita, I've come to accept the fact that I'm not going to live to be an old man." But he sort of put it in terms of maybe ten years. I think the closest he ever got to saying it was when he said to me, "Maybe I have five years." Cliff never got to the point where he said, "I know that I'm dying." We never got to say that. There were many reasons for that. A lot of it had to do with the way death happened for him.

I thought this whole experience would kill me. There was a long time when I didn't think I could live. Truly. Now that I have, and now that I am five years beyond Cliff's death, I can say that it was one of the most awesome experiences I've ever had. Not that I'd want to repeat it. But the person I've become—the changes, the growth—have been amazing. I certainly don't know it all. God, I'll run out of time and I will still not have gotten it all. I know that. But it's been an incredible experience. It is truly a gift to walk that walk with someone. It's one of the most intimate experiences of life. You're never the same. I don't know how anybody who has really been there, done this, could ever be the same again.

I had been so enmeshed with Cliff that it was as though my own life were in danger, watching him die. Having him go through death, I don't know how else to say it except that somehow, emotionally, I went through it, too. We were both afraid and kind of hanging on, but we were sure that we were in charge of what was happening. The truth is, we never were in charge. We never, ever were. So I had to break. And I did. When I say it broke me, it did. It broke me in two. I think the choice for me then was, am I going to stay down there, broken?

That experience took me down to a place I'd never been. I've never been lower or deeper in my life. I realized that I could stay broken or try to get up and be mended and be stronger. And when I did get up, I was indeed all of those things. I was a better person. Not that I'll never be afraid in my life again, or not that I'll never want to be in control again. But now I have different eyes. I have a different heart. It was like a rebirth for me. I didn't leave all the negative things behind. But you know what? The ones I didn't leave behind, I've looked in the eye. And if I still carry them, I know they're there, and they'll never be a part of me like they were a part of me in my younger years. They have their place. But I'm a different person.

I went through the Hospice grief work twice. During that second time, there was an intern doing a residency with Hospice. She was a lovely young woman who was into Native American culture and dance therapy. That's the kind of thing she brought to our group. This young woman came to my house one day and did a little smudging ceremonial at the house. Cliff's presence was still so present that she felt that it might be helpful to come and do what the American Indians do to help a spirit move on. So she burned a tight pack of herbs tied with a string on the bottom. We had a whole ceremony, just the two of us. She walked through the house with the burning herbs. She went to all the corners of the house and the bedroom.

I was not so sure that what she was doing was necessary. It didn't seem problematic to me to have Cliff around. I mean, I wasn't seeing him sitting in the chair or anything. But I was keenly aware that I felt his presence. Oh, a couple of times, I guess I sort of saw something. Cliff died his own way, and he was going to leave in his own his time. I don't think the smudging was going to impress him that much. And I don't remember any dramatic change from what she did. I think it simply made others feel better. Cliff's presence was okay with me. I knew these things would run their course.

I don't feel Cliff in the house any more now. I remember the time when that changed. I walked into this house, and he wasn't here. It wasn't the same anymore. But I carry Cliff inside me. He is as much a part of my life today as he was when we were married, just in a different way. That's a gift and an incredible comfort. People told me that the time would come when this would happen, when you make the person you lose a part of you. Initially, you can't hear that kind of information. But it did happen.

It feels confusing when I think, How could each one of us still be present? Trillions of human beings have been born and have died. How could each one continue? I don't know. Maybe we all become one collective energy source. I don't know. But I know it doesn't end. I mean, somebody's still guiding me. I am so in touch with that now that sometimes it stops me in my tracks. And it makes me smile. It's like I see stardust falling down on me from above that's saying, "Nita, do it this way; do it that way; do it." I'm not playing a part in it. Of that I am sure.

I kept Cliff's ashes for a long time, too. Then we went down to the coast and put them in the ocean on the Cape. I went with his parents and his sister, but I kept a little bit of Cliff's ashes for myself. I needed to be able to have a moment alone to sprinkle his ashes myself. So I went back to the Cape to do that, alone. It was pouring rain that day. There were seals. I'd never seen them there before. One of the seals left the others and stayed with me the entire time. The seal was in the water, very close to the shore, *very* close. And it didn't surprise me. When all the other seals had left—and they all went in the same direction—this one didn't join them. I could see his head, his eyes. He just bobbed there.

And I remember doing the ashes. I've never been one for knowing much which way the wind was blowing or not blowing. I had a raincoat on, and it was soaking wet. When I let the ashes go, they blew back onto my raincoat. They stuck on. So I walked back to the car with Cliff's ashes on me. I thought, it's a good thing his family isn't here to see this.

I think Cliff and I will see each other again. I often think of a line in a Carly Simon song. I first heard it after Cliff's death. She sings, "There's more room in a broken heart. Don't feel bad for me. There's more room in a broken heart." And I often thought, you know, Cliff was the love of my life, and I will love again. I have loved, and I will love again. There is so much room in a heart, and maybe there is more room in a broken one. Maybe that's why they break.

Amy Silverberg

Amy Silverberg, a teacher, counselor, and retired minister, was with her baby, Sharon, at the child's death. When I met with her, Amy told me how significantly her life was redefined by Sharon's birth and, again, by the child's death. Sharon's presence in Amy's life taught Amy a kind of strength that she said she previously hadn't known.

When my daughter, Sharon, was born, that was a revelation in and of itself. I already had two healthy boys, and then I had Sharon. In those days, you had a baby and then the hospital staff took it away and you didn't see it until they finally brought it back to you. I will never forget when the nurse brought Sharon in to me for the first time. She was the first girl in my life. Initially, I wanted to have five boys. That was my goal, five boys. But there I was, alone in the room, and the nurse carried Sharon in, handed me the bundle of baby and blankets, and left again. I held Sharon gently, cradling her, caring for her neck, expecting her to be limp like a baby. But she pushed against my shoulder with her hands. She put her hands on me and pushed herself back so far that she didn't even have my hand behind her neck. She looked me square in the eyes. Babies' eyes usually go wandering in all directions, but Sharon stared at me directly, wide eyed and smiling, and then she crumpled like a baby. The smile she gave me was one of a radiant recognition. It was like she was saying, "Yes, I found you. I did good!"

My experience with Sharon was a gift, a gift from her to me, a total experience unlike anything I'd ever known. I had been a very insecure person for most of my life, never really sure that anybody liked me. "Why," I asked, "would they?" My feelings were part of a battered-child syndrome. But then there was this infant saying to me, "You're it! You're it, and I'm so glad I'm here with you. You're it." In the hospital where I gave birth, Sharp Hospital in San Diego, staff actually graded the babies. They awarded Sharon an A+. In her bassinet, in the nursery, she was up on her elbows looking around, at less than twenty-four hours of age. I mean, she was *vital,* full of energy, eyes tracking. In the photo they took of her in the hospital, she was bright eyed, looking out at the world.

From the very first moment she was born, she and I were communicating. One of the first things she learned to do was imitate me. I would go "click, click, click" with my tongue, and she picked that up, in her first month. She would greet me that way when I came in in the morning or when she wanted some attention. Unlike the boys, by the time I brought Sharon home, she was sleeping through the night, at three and a half, four days old. She didn't ever cry. She never cried. She had her way, "click, click, click," to get attention. She knew she was going to get attention. Even the boys couldn't keep their hands off her. I'd hear one of them say, "Hey, it's my turn to hold her." This child was loved!

By the time she reached two and a half months, however, I realized something was radically wrong. Sharon was strong when she was born, but by two and a half months, she had yet to roll over. She could no longer get up on her elbows. I took her in to the doctor and he spent an hour and a half going over her, neurologically, spending time with her, seeing what her reactions and responses were. The doctor finally came up with a list of five possibilities of what might be going on with her. The options were all ugly. One possibility was an early onset of multiple sclerosis. One was muscular dystrophy. With both of those diseases, she could live into her twenties and maybe thirties. Another disease the doctor suspected was Werdnig-Hoffmann disease. It's a genetic congenital disorder. It turned out to be what Sharon had.

If I had married anybody else, or my husband had married anybody else, we wouldn't have had it. But together we produced it.

For families that produce it, there's a 50 percent possibility for every pregnancy that you're going to have it.

There was no way of knowing right away what Sharon had. None of the things that the doctor enumerated for me, none of the possibilities, were diagnosable at that point. We had to wait and see. Sharon was born on St. Patrick's Day. We went through the summer, and she was not getting better. She was going very slowly downhill. She was still making strong eye contact with me, always. And conversing with me, going, "click, click, click" with me, always. There was a sense that she was talking to me. There was a sense that we communicated together. "Hi, how are you, Darling?" "I'm fine. How are you, Mom?" It was not on a baby level. There was mature intelligence in her, and I knew it. But I've always felt that about babies. I always feel a brand-new infant is the closest we get to God. A brand-new infant anything, even a puppy. That's why we're so attracted to infants. I believe that.

On Labor Day weekend, Sharon went into crisis and had to go into the hospital. I didn't recognize her. We had taken her on our vacation to Arrow Head, a mountainous place east of Los Angeles. It's at six thousand feet, and that stressed Sharon's breathing abilities. But it happened slowly. It's like somebody can look at you and say, "Oh my, you're going gray," when you haven't noticed it really because you've been *going* gray. I didn't see it, but I took her to the hospital. It was the Friday of the beginning of Labor Day weekend that she went into the hospital. That was a terrible time. We thought we were losing her. I wanted to be there for her meals—a bottle only. It was a good thing that she was used to a bottle. She was accustomed to that from the start, and at the end, by seven and a half months, when she died, she could not have done anything but a bottle. There was no way.

We brought her home finally. I begged the pediatrician. He had only seen Werdnig-Hoffmann disease twice before. One in five hundred thousand babies gets it. It's a very rare thing. It's an infantile syndrome like Lou Gehrig's disease. Medical researchers know very little about it. There's no way to stop it, and there's very little doctors can do for it. If you've got it, you've got it and you're going to die from it, and that's it.

While Sharon was in the hospital, I got up early in the mornings to set things out for breakfast for everybody. Then I left, drove to the hospital, which was a half hour away, was there with Sharon for breakfast, lunch, and dinner. Then I came home, fixed dinner for the family, and tried to be a mother for two little boys. It was a terror of a time, just a terror. So for four days I did this, and it seemed like four months. It was just forever. I finally said to the doctor, "Isn't there some way we can get an oxygen tent that I can rent?" There wasn't a rentable oxygen tent anywhere in the world. We couldn't find one. No one would give it up. This was 1962. But then I turned to the muscular dystrophy organization. The organization refused to rent a tent to me. They insisted on giving it to me for as long as I needed it. Guess who I still give money to? So we brought Sharon home. But the oxygen tent put a surface between us. I couldn't hold her.

Two weeks before Sharon died, she lost the ability to move. One week before she died, she refused anything in terms of nourishment. She only took the bottle that had water with the medication in it that kept her gut settled. I said to my husband, "I think she's saying good-bye. I expect that she'll go." But the process felt long and drawn out; she could have lasted till New Year's. As far as I was concerned, it could have gone on forever. Sharon was just amazing. Each week, the doctor would come. One week he said to me, "I wish for just a little strychnine, just a little, to put her out of her misery, but I can't do it. It's against the law. I can't do it." For an animal going through that kind of struggle, you would definitely put an animal down. You can't do that with your child. You can't do it with your parent.

One week after Sharon stopped taking nourishment, I went in with the bottle, first thing in the morning—well, I had gone in earlier and changed her diaper. But now her brother, Stevie, had gone off to his kindergarten, and her brother, Rick, was down the street playing with a friend. My husband was at work. Everybody else had scattered.

I went in and I picked Sharon up and had her in my arms. The room was long and narrow. I was sitting at one end. Kitty-corner from me was the window in the room. It was a big window, rectangular and big for the room, which was not a big room. I was sitting facing the window with Sharon in my arms. I went to offer her the bottle. She was looking up at my eyes, just this little limp baby. It was like holding a Raggedy Ann doll. There was no strength to her, no weight to her. She was almost a skeleton at that point. And all of a sudden, her entire body began to resonate with energy. I could feel it. It wasn't an electric shock, but I could feel it in her body.

Then Sharon turned. She shifted her whole body in my arms and looked out the window. The expression on her face was absolute, total bliss. Total radiance. And she turned back to me, having taken in just this gaspy, joyful intake of air, this kind of "Ah, ah, ah"—I don't know how to describe that in words—and looked at me, and that was her last breath. The look on her face was as if she was saying, "Can you see it, Mom?" And she was gone. It's thirty-seven years later and I still get goose bumps remembering it. She was gone.

But for that ten-second period that it took her to shift, turn, look, acknowledge, she was briefly alive and well. She had become vital again. My sense was that she was filled with sight and sound of something beyond my vision that was so joyous that it was like, "Oh, this is where I'm going. Yippee. Can you see it Mom? It's neat." And she was gone.

When she took that last breath, all the life went out of the Raggedy Ann doll, and she was just at peace. There was a sense of peace to it. I sat there for probably fifteen minutes with her in my arms, acknowledging that she was gone. It was her last breath, and she was gone. And her last breath was simply to take in the joy, if you will. I've never thought of it like that, but that breath, that blissful breath, was to animate the soul so that it could leave.

I've never seen anything like this. It was unique—absolutely, flat out. In those minutes I sat there holding her, I was feeling the emptiness. When you give so much of yourself to any project or person, and then it's gone—I don't care what it is—you're going to feel a void in your life.

So I was feeling that sense of "Now, what do I do with myself? What's my purpose now?" Then I realized that I had to let people know, and I didn't want to have to go through that. I cried, yet at that point, I was relatively at peace with having her gone. But to have to share that experience was not something I was ready to do. It took me months before I could talk about it.

Sharon came to me, I am convinced, to give me the gift of myself, of self-knowledge that I didn't have, and to shift me off the path that I was walking on a spiritual level. This process with Sharon regrouped my thinking, got me back to my original belief system, the one I was born with. I got a better education in religion as a result of her coming and going than you'd get in a theological school. After her death, I studied religious belief systems about dying with a vengeance. I realized there wasn't any one religious belief system in which I believed. All of them had something, but none of them had it all. All that study turned me around completely, away from the church I was attending and into metaphysics, into natural healing. The whole searching process I went through was as a result of Sharon's coming and going. To this day, I probably would be a matron fixing the flowers for the Episcopal church, wherever I was living, if it hadn't been for Sharon.

There's no way that a child comes into your life and within hours of birth, looks at you with recognition. With recognition. There's no question in my mind, Sharon knew who I was and it was a deliberate move—on her part—that she was in my arms. There was just that sense of "This is right." There was intelligence in that move. There was an acknowledgment of me as well as of herself in that gesture of hers.

Eyes are the doorway to the soul. So to connect, soul to soul, as we did in the hospital, was a deliberate move on her part. Sharon pushed away from me, back and spine rigid, eyes on my eyes and just a shudder of joy. You can't tell me she didn't come from somewhere on purpose, and if that's true, when she left, she left recognizing the Holy Ghost in everybody else, the choirs of God, angels, whatever you want to call it, even if it was simply a guide that she recognized. I don't know. In that moment, to me, there was an orchestra playing and horns blowing and angels' wings flopping around. There should have been feathers on the floor when Sharon left. That's what she gave to me. She filled me with a knowledge of what she saw, without my having seen it. It was just glorious.

And with an experience like that, there's an imperative that you rethink your beliefs about birthing and dying. Where do we come from? We come from somewhere. Where do we go? We go somewhere. We're not gone, and we weren't gone before we got here. And if that's true, then reincarnation makes ultimate sense.

Sharon has taught me about dying. It's been an inner knowing that keeps blossoming. It's like the lotus opening. You glean something new, get a specific interest in it. You get more and more interested and you learn more and more and more and you grow. It's beautiful. Sharon knocked me off the road of "Mommy." "Wife." "These are my obligations." "This is what I have to do with my life, whether I like it or not." "This is where I'm going." "This is who I am." It was Sharon who planted the seed that I had to start learning for myself something other than what I believed life was about. I had to get some answers that didn't come from other people's belief systems. It was Sharon's life and her death that gave me that gift, that gave me a true understanding of who I really am.

Ann Schauffler

I had had a casual acquaintanceship with preschool teacher and artist Ann Schauffler for years, but not until I began to collect people's stories for this book did I get to know her more fully. In her home in suburban Boston, she shared with me her story about her mother's death. Her story is not only one of death, family, and acceptance but also one of intuition and trust. Ann, her husband, and I have developed a close friendship since that initial afternoon in her house, and my life has been deeply enriched as a result.

My mother had been confronted with cancer ever since I was in college. When I was in college in the late sixties, she had melanoma on one of her retinas one spring and had to have that eye surgically removed. Because my parents were living in Europe at the time, I didn't hear about it until after it all happened. She wrote to tell me from the hospital that the day before, she'd had surgery.

My mother never talked about that stuff. I think part of that reason was because *her* mother died of cancer. Most of my mother's growing up was spent with her own mother in and out of various cancer situations. My mother's father committed suicide when she was thirteen, and she was left to be with her mother who was still in the throes of cancer. I think it was from her mother that my mom got the sort of stoic attitude, "Life goes on. I'm doing this but I don't want it to upset my kids."

So that was the first bout my mother had with cancer. Then in 1971 she got breast cancer and had a radical mastectomy. That time,

I found out the day before the surgery. We have a family history of not informing each other, of not wanting to upset anybody. But I ended up getting on a plane and going to see her. My parents were then living in Washington, D.C. On the phone my dad had hesitated to tell me because he knew my husband was doing his final project in the theater department at Yale Drama School and my father didn't want to upset him or throw the project off. When my mother was in recovery in the hospital, I said to her then, "You cannot exclude us from these things in your life. We need to be a part of it. We're all family. You have to promise me that you'll never do that again." So she was good about that in the following years.

She survived the breast cancer and did fine. She had some leftover discomfort, but nothing major. Then in 1982 she found out she had lung cancer in the middle lobe of her right lung. She had the lobe removed and had to go through radiation. She was forty-nine when she had her breast cancer. In 1982 she was sixty. Then only two years later, she was diagnosed with cancer in her other lung, in the lower part of one of the lobes. She came up to Boston to have surgery. One of my brothers was living in Boston, as was I, and another brother was in Maine. She wanted my dad to be able to be near family so they found a surgeon at Mass. General. We all sort of rallied around. She had surgery then to remove a section of her lung. She was on some drugs, but she didn't do any chemo. That must have been in 1984. Then a year or so later more cancer was diagnosed. It was a different kind of cancer. It wasn't localized. It was very webby in her lungs. The only way to treat it was through chemo, so she decided to do that.

My parents had to commute to where she was getting the chemo. It was a day-long trip, and she would get violently ill on the way home. She started taking the drug that would prevent the nausea and the sickness, but she also started sleeping a lot, sometimes for two days at a time. She would have chemo, and that would be like a one-week ordeal, and then she'd be all right for a couple of weeks and then it would be time to go back to chemo again. She was determined to get through it. She was really strong that way. We came together a lot as a family, as much as we could. She felt very good about the care she was getting. She was frustrated as hell that it was happening, but she thought she needed to give it everything she had, to get better. She was invested in her family, her husband, and her life and was determined to keep going. After six months there was no significant change in the cancer. At that point, my mother decided that the quality of her life was so diminished by having to go through the chemo and losing days from the knockout drug to keep her from being sick that she just decided to stop and to live as long as she could, feeling good.

After that, my mother got very involved with MADRE, an international women's human-rights organization that works in partnership with women's community-based groups in conflict areas worldwide. MADRE is designed to provide an alternative to war and violence through a people-to-people exchange of direct relief and understanding.

My youngest brother, Richard, who was involved in a lot of social action in San Francisco, started telling her about MADRE, and she became really interested in it. At the time, MADRE was strongest in Nicaragua/Central America, where there were many "disappearances" of sons, husbands, and uncles because of the U.S.-sponsored contra war. My mother got as much information about MADRE as she could, and she sent money. She corresponded with the organization's office in New York. She closely related to those women in Central America who had lost their husbands and sons. She felt it very personally.

As my mother aged, she became much more liberal politically. My father was in the Navy, a career officer in the Navy, and they were staunch Republicans. But as she got older, it was easier to talk to her—she came to her senses! Richard was really involved in some radical stuff out in California—Marxist movements. My mother really wanted to understand why he was taking groups to Cuba and why he was going to Nicaragua. She had total respect for her children's decisions about what they did in their lives. My dad was a little taken aback, but he supported her involvement in it. She was sort of an anomaly down in Florida, the person who supported Planned Parenthood. She finally found another woman or two who were at least into Planned Parenthood and to whom she could relate.

My parents were living in Daytona Beach when she was dealing with lung cancer and also when she became interested in MADRE. At that point, her health was fairly good. She'd lost her hair during chemo. She said of all the things she had had to endure, that that particular loss was the hardest. It had been a shock for her to lose her eye. She was a very visual person and an artist. She did painting and design, but she learned to compensate for that. She could still see as keenly with one eye as some people never learn to see with two. Then losing a breast was hard. She was a strikingly beautiful woman. The eye loss was very apparent. The breast you could kind of cover up some. But she said losing the hair was the worst part. She would sleep with a turban. She wouldn't even let my dad see her without any hair; she was mortified by it. She was wearing these "G.D. wigs," as she called them. And finally, finally she started getting some hair growth and she was so excited. She tossed the wigs in the air. She sent them off for the grandchildren to use in their dress-up boxes. She was so glad to get rid of them.

She had diminished capacity to breathe because of the lung cancer, so she had to give up a lot of physical activities. She didn't really exert herself, physically. But she was determined to go when MADRE decided to have a first annual conference in New York City. She was there for a week. They later told me how she just walked in. There she was by herself and she said, "Well, what can I do?" They had her setting up different kinds of exhibits and making flower arrangements. She knew it was a risk to go to a big city like that, to expose herself to possibly getting sick. She was more susceptible than usual because of her diminished lung capacity.

The doctor had apparently told her, "The cancer probably won't kill you for a while, but if you get any kind of bronchial infection or pneumonia, that may be it." So she wore gloves when she was on the subway. She was careful that way. But she didn't want to stop. When she got off the train in Boston, when I picked her up, she was beaming. She said it was the most fantastic experience of her life, to be in a room full of women with this common connection and this common interest. She said the energy and power and commitment and community was so exciting. She was just flying. It was her first real experience like that. Going there by herself, she was so proud.

She and my dad stayed with us for a couple of days, and she

started to kind of feel this ache in her shoulder. She worried about metastases. Anytime she felt an ache, she admitted she worried. But she passed off the ache in the shoulder. She was an optimist. She would sit there and rub her shoulder, but she thought that maybe she'd carried too many heavy things in New York. Shortly after that, she and my dad went out to Cape Cod for a visit. They were there for about five days. We talked to them when they first got out there to make sure everything was okay. It was the end of the school year, and with all the activity here, we weren't really in touch until I got a phone call from my father who said, "Ann, your mom hasn't been feeling well, and I think we need to get her to a doctor." I said, "Do you want to do it out there, or do you want to come back here," and he said, "I think we need to come back with you." I said, "How bad is it?" And he said, "I think she may have pneumonia. She's had fever and chills and can't seem to shake it." He was distraught. So I said, "We'll be there."

My husband and I borrowed my brother's van. We brought blankets and pillows and all kinds of other supplies. They wanted us to come and get them. We left the next morning and got there before noon. My dad was white as a ghost. He was practically in tears. He said, "This isn't good. This isn't good." I told him it was okay; we were there. We'd help.

We went in to see my mom. She looked at me and said, "I really don't feel well." And I said, "I know. We're here to take you to the hospital. Is there anything I can do for you now?" And she said "I don't know." I said, "Well, would you like me to bathe you?" She said, "Oh, that would be so wonderful. I haven't had a bath. I haven't been able to get out of bed."

That bath was an amazing thing. It was sort of a beginning for me, bathing my mother as she lay in bed with a totally exposed body. It was such a powerful connection. It was symbolic of so much of the mother-daughter relationship. Here I was, bathing her like she used to bathe me. We had a really strong relationship. Yet I felt like that bath was the most intimate moment I had had with her. I sponge bathed her, her whole body. I remember she took the washcloth and washed between her legs herself. Then I dressed her in a clean nightgown and said, "We brought the van so you can put the seat back.

We have blankets for you." She said, "Good. Just get me to the hospital as soon as you can."

We carried her out to the car and put her on the front seat and extended it back. We had pillows and blankets and water. She hadn't eaten anything in about three days. She hadn't been able to eat. And we just drove. We drove straight from South Yarmouth to Emerson Hospital in Concord. That was the nearest hospital to my home. I didn't want to get lost in Mass. General. That turned out to be a good decision. We got to the hospital about 4:00 P.M., my dad and I and Rob, my husband at the time. Rob had lost his wife to cancer when he was about twenty-eight. Rob was a real comfort to my dad. He understood the emotions that were going on with Dad. I felt as if I was totally connected to my mom.

At the hospital, the person taking her history asked my mother about her parents and what they had died of. Her mother had died of cancer. Then the woman asked, "And your father?" My mother paused. Then she looked at me and said, "a gunshot wound," staring into my eyes. That confession was a major one. It had taken so long for her to tell us about this suicide. This was the first time I had been present when she had been asked that question by someone outside the family. It seemed that she was still guarding "the family secret" yet revealing a bit of the truth. That moment, when she looked into my eyes, was about her struggle with her father's death. It was about love and trust and survival. It was about our connection.

We had to wait a couple of hours before they got her upstairs. They did X-rays. She had pneumonia. So they moved her to a room that had oxygen and they tried to make her comfortable. We could put her on antibiotics, but the doctor wasn't sure that anything could help because of her diminished lung capacity. My mother was still quite awake. Because it was near dinnertime, she wanted everybody to go home and have dinner with the kids. She didn't want the kids to be worried that we weren't there. She wanted us all to leave.

She always had to be in control, and she was determined to control this, too. She said, "No, really, I'll be fine. I promised the doctors that I'd be fine. I've got the medication. It's really important for you to go. I want you all to be together for dinner." So very reluctantly, we left. Since we only lived about twenty minutes away, I guess we thought, Okay, we can do this. We're close by. So my brother's family and their kids and my kids, we all got together and had dinner. Everybody was distracted. We were trying to get Dad to relax and tell us what had happened. He said, "She got sick. I don't know if she's going to make it." And I said, "Well, do you feel like you want to go back to the hospital? What should we do?" And he said, "I don't know. I don't know what to do."

At about 10:00 P.M., we got a call from the doctor at the hospital who was tending her. He said, "I think you'd better come back. She's not doing well at all. You'd better come back." So my dad and I headed over. We went in, and she wasn't conscious at that point. Her eyes were closed, and she didn't know we were there. She couldn't open her eyes, and she was breathing hard. The doctor said to my dad, "Things are pretty serious. What do you want to have happen if she needs resuscitating?" Dad said, "Nothing. We have Living Wills. We don't want any resuscitation."

The doctor said, "I'm really sorry. I'm really sorry." He reached out and touched both of us. He was very kind. We went into the room and I said to Dad, "We need to talk to Mom. Even though she can't talk back, she may be hearing us, so we need to talk to her. Why don't you talk to her? I'll step out and let you talk to her. And then I'll come back in." So I left him for a few minutes, but soon he came and got me, saying, "Annie, please come in." So I did. He was uncomfortable and just so upset. They had a deeply loving relationship. They were incredibly close. They had had an enviable, wonderful life together, very romantic and so entwined.

I went over to her. I was stroking her head. I told her that we were there and that we loved her. I told her that Rob and Fred and Richard were all sending their love. I said that we were going to be with her, that Dad and I were going to stay with her. I told her how much I loved her and what a wonderful mother she'd been. I told her that I had had so many wonderful things in my life because of her. I told her the grandchildren loved her. But the most important thing I wanted to tell her was that we were going to be there.

To me, that was such an honor, to be able to be with her. When her own mother was dying, my mother was pregnant with me. Because my mother had had two or three miscarriages before me, doctors would not let her travel during her pregnancies. So she never got back to see her mother before her mother died. Her mother died two weeks before I was born. That meant that my mother wasn't even able to go to her own mother's funeral. She didn't go back to her hometown until I was about six weeks old. She never voiced it, but I always felt it was a very difficult time in her life, to be faced with the birth of a child at the same time as the death of her mother. I remember talking to her about it once and saying it must have been so hard. And she could barely talk about it.

My conviction was, I've got to be with my mother when she dies. I always feared that because they lived so far away and because of her inability to tell me what was going on, I might not have that chance. I was afraid I was not going to know. So it was powerful to be in that room during that time. I was incredibly thankful for it. She must have been, too, whether or not she could voice it.

My father looked across the bed at me and said, "What do we do now?" and I said, "We're going to sit here, and we're going to talk." And I said, "Let's let Mom listen to us." We started telling family stories, remembering things that had happened. I was asking him about things he and Mom had done. It was really good but it also was hard because nobody else was there. The nurse would come in periodically and check her. My mother was clearly getting uncomfortable. We said to the nurse, "Please, keep her comfortable. You've got to give her something." My mother seemed to be in pain. She was making noises and then her body was tensing up. It was clear she was suffering. She couldn't have morphine. She was deathly allergic to morphine, but she could have Demerol.

"Bring in the Demerol. Just keep her calm," we said. "There's no reason why she should have to feel anything." We asked the nurses, "What is happening?" They really had no answers, but it was clear that it was just a matter of time. They said, "She seems comfortable now." "She still has a low-grade fever." "Her lungs are very full." "There's no way of telling what's going to happen."

Dad needed to have some kind of framework—something. I explained to him, "You can't predict it, Dad." Every now and then, we'd tell Mom we loved her. Then there came a point where it seemed like she really was struggling more to breathe. Maybe this was after a couple of hours. I said to Dad, "You know, I think maybe we need to give her permission to go. Sometimes a person who is dying really needs to hear that it's okay, that everybody's going to be okay." He said, "I can't do that." And I said, "Well, do you want me to?" And he said, "Yeah."

So I leaned over and I talked into her ear and I said, "We're all loving you. Thank you for all the beautiful things you've done for us. We want you to know that it's okay. You can go. It's okay. We'll all be together." My dad had to leave the room. He couldn't take it. When he came back, I asked him about his fondest memories. He talked about how for the past two Christmases they'd gone out to the desert in California and spent time in a friend's house. They drove around through the desert looking at all the flowers and seeing wild sheep.

He talked about how beautiful it was. He talked about Aunt Marion, his great-aunt who was sort of like our grandmother because we didn't know any of our grandparents when we were growing up. Aunt Marion was an artist and she used to go west and paint the desert in the spring. My father and I were laughing. He started relaxing and in a way was able to laugh about some of the silly stuff that had happened, camping trips that we'd taken as kids and stuff like that. There would be moments when we'd turn and look at Mom as she tried to breathe. We were stroking her hand the whole time, and Dad was holding her hand. We were stroking her leg. We were always in physical contact with her. We never let go.

At first I was very conscious of the fact that we were in half of a hospital room. There was somebody on the other side of the curtain, a much older woman. I didn't know anything about her, who she was or anything. It was quiet. It was late at night. Mom was probably asleep the whole time. After a while, the surroundings became irrelevant. I felt like the energy was all focused on Mom's bed and on the three of us there together. I became more aware of our physical relationship to each other and our spiritual relationship to each other. That was the strongest thing there. All of a sudden it didn't seem like we had had enough time together. I just wished my mother had been awake so we could have had those last words while her eyes were open. I do feel like she heard us. I don't know how much she heard of our reminiscing, but I know she heard us. We were right there by her ear.

Then, as we were talking—I can't even remember what we were talking about—while Dad was holding Mom's hand and I had my hand on her leg, all of a sudden I felt this kind of—I just had this physical sensation; it was just like tingling, total tingling all through my body, from my toes and out through my head. It just sort of stopped me. I just remember really being taken aback by it, and I looked over at Mom and I said, "Dad." Then Mom took four really long breaths. I remember it was four. I was thinking they were for her four children. I was holding my dad's hand and I was touching Mom. We were like a triangle. And then she just stopped. We looked at her. And she started breathing again. We couldn't move. Finally there was another big sigh and a big breath in. And then silence. We sat there. Dad started crying, and I started crying. He leaned over and held her body. I lay my head on her lap.

That night, I felt as if the three of us had been there at my birth and the three of us were there at her death. It was back to the original threesome. It was an honored place to be. I felt like I was really sharing an extraordinary moment with my parents. My dad was really depending on me to help him through it. He was very verbal about that: "I'm glad you're here. I'm glad you know what you're doing, because I don't." The intimacy was amazing, unique. It was unlike any other time in life. You're also trying everything you can to be able to let go, knowing that you've got to let go but you don't want to. That struggle is going on. I actually felt like I had settled that issue more than my dad had at the time. I just felt, I know this is what we have to do. Okay, this is it. This is the time. We are here.

I had always wondered if I would be strong enough to do it, if I could do it, but I felt like once I was there, I wasn't afraid of it. It seemed like this was just the part of what had to happen. Her death was really more peaceful than I had imagined. Her body looked peaceful and serene. All the struggle was gone from her face. As I was standing there, I was struck by the realization, She's not here any more. This is not *her*. This is just the body that she occupied. But she's not here.

My father went over and took off her ring. I was amazed because it just slipped off her finger. It was the ring she had had on ever since her mother had died. She wore it all the time. She never, ever took it off. I later found out that one of the times they were in the desert she'd gone to a jeweler. She couldn't remove the ring. She had the jeweler cut it off and make it larger so that it could be slipped off later on. Then he took off the engagement ring, and the nurse said, "Do you want the wedding ring?" and he said, "No, I don't. I want her to keep it." He later said the same thing at the funeral home.

We stayed with Mom for a while, and then Dad said, "I think I have to leave." I kissed her. She was still a little warm. I don't know long it takes for the body to cool down, but there was still warmth there. Her smell was still there, just sort of lingering. I left Dad alone in the room with her for a while. He was in there for about ten minutes, just crying. He needed to do that privately, to be with her and hold onto her. They'd been married forty-four years. They were each other's salvation. Then I went in. I put my arm around him. We talked about how strange it was that her body was there and she wasn't. It felt like we were looking at some sort of case of a human form. We talked about how beautiful she looked and what a beautiful body she had inhabited. My father was saying, "I can't believe it. This is so hard." We talked a little about having tried to prepare ourselves for it, over the years, but now that it had really happened, it was so painful.

But I felt okay about it. I didn't feel wracked with harsh grief. I felt like it had been an honor, such an honorable experience to be there with her. I was also thankful that she wasn't still in pain and that she didn't have to go through a long, prolonged death. It was relatively short and sweet, her dying. There was something very comforting about seeing her body at such peace.

I was struck with my mother's last breaths. I remember those moments being really powerful. I'd read about it. Then I witnessed it. When the last breaths started to happen, I had a sense of, Oh, *this* is what happens. I was really moved by how the body just kind of fills up with air and then lets go. It's a release, almost a yoga sort of thing, in a strange way. You know, when you're starting to meditate, how you take breaths sort of to calm yourself? I hope that I die in a blissful state like that, too. It's definitely an amazing thing.

When my brother arrived from Maine, we went back to the hospital so he could see Mom. There was still this amazing serenity and peacefulness to her. He sat with her for a while. Later on that day, we went to the funeral home. My dad told the funeral director, "I don't want you to do anything to her. She's beautiful; please don't put on makeup. She didn't wear makeup. Just let her be." When we came back with my brothers, the mortician had wrapped her in a white sheet. She was lying in a box, and she looked beautiful. The four of us stood there, and my dad came in with us. We each had separate moments with this body. We talked about how she wasn't there. She looked very peaceful. There was something remarkable about that peacefulness. The body wasn't feeling anything anymore. You just knew that there was a release from physical pain, there was no physicalness any more. I really understood what *soul* meant when we looked at a body like that. I totally understood what *soul* meant.

We had a family memorial service about a week later with a couple of very close friends. We had all of the kids, spouses, grandchildren, from ages four up, I think my daughter, Jess, was the oldest at that point, at sixteen. We formed a circle and sat. Richard and I had gone to a florist in the next town, and we had gathered together this incredible bouquet of flowers, her favorites as well as flowers from every region in which my parents had lived. We had birds of paradise. We had iris. Each of the grandchildren had brought a flower from his or her own garden to put in the vase, too. Everybody had had a week to think about it and prepare what they wanted to say.

My daughter, Jess, had written something. But she was in tears the whole time. She couldn't even speak. So her grandfather said, "That's okay, Jess, it's really okay." My nephew wrote a poem, and his sister played the flute. My son was four. He had drawn some pictures, so he held up his pictures and showed them. Everybody had something to contribute. We made it into a book later on. We reproduced it for everybody in the family and for some close friends who couldn't be there. I did a drawing of the bouquet for the book.

About a year later, there was a memorial service for Cousin Ann who had died. I remember sitting there feeling blessed by the presence of something. I felt like my mother and Cousin Ann were somehow there for me, and I felt like I was being showered with love. All of a sudden I had this feeling that everything was going to be okay, that I was going to be okay, I was going to make it.

Being with my mother in those final moments has made me more aware of my relationship with my daughter, Jess. She was sixteen at the time, but since then, we've grown more and more close. We talk about everything together. I know I'm much more open with my daughter than my mother was with me. All the things I wish my mother had been able to talk to me about, I talk to Jess about. That's really good, a tight connection, and I know she'll be there for me, and that would be lovely if we could be together when it's my time to die.

After my mother's death, my father kept having visits from her. I'd call him up and I'd say, "How are you doing?" He'd say, "I'm fine. I'm fine. I'm playing golf." And I'd say, "No, *how* are you doing, Dad? What has it been like for you?" Then he would tell me. He'd say, "You're going to think I'm crazy, but I think your mother was here last night. I was almost asleep and I really felt this weight on the bed." He would tell me about these kinds of things and about his dreams. I could reassure him that all these things were good, they were normal, and they were beautiful. Those dreams must have been comforting for him. I kept thinking, "How come I don't get those kinds of visits? She must be spending all her time with him." I really only had about two or three dreams with my mom in them. Dad still says he dreams about her every single night. He's just afraid to tell his second wife. He doesn't want her to feel that he's cheating on her because he keeps "seeing" Mom.

Three years ago, my younger brother, Rob, committed suicide. Rob was two years my junior. He and I had been estranged because of some stupid argument. He would not give in, and I was tired of trying to break through. So we hadn't really spoken to each other for a while. Rob really suffered a lot when my mom died. He felt she was the glue that held everything together, and after her death, he felt that everything was falling apart. He was having a lot of problems in his personal life. His marriage had fallen apart. But the comforting thought for everybody was that my mother and Rob were together. My dad kept saying, "The only way I can even begin to try to accept this is to think your mom and brother are together. They're connected. They're up there."

I had a real physical reaction when Rob died—not knowing at that moment that he had died. My husband, Stan, and I were taking a walk with two of our children, Margaret and Sasha. All of a sudden I had an excruciating pain in my body. It doubled me over, and I had to stop. Stan and the kids were walking way ahead, and finally they turned around and saw me and came back. I said, "I can't walk. I've got to sit down." It was like my breath was gone. I had a pain that felt like a knife in my torso. I was sitting on a bench, trying to get my breath. Stan said, "Should I go get the car?" I said, "No, I think I can make it, but I may have to go slowly." And I did. I had to stop a couple more times. I was practically doubled over.

By the time we got to the house, I said, "I can't sit up. I have to go lie down." I thought maybe I was having a gastric attack, which I'd never had in my life before. And Stan said, "Why don't you take some Pepto-Bismol?" I did and went to lie down, but I was in tremendous pain, incredible pain. I couldn't get up. The pain was under my ribs. I was out, flat on my back. I couldn't move, couldn't do anything. I was in tears. I didn't know what was going on.

Later that night, about 2:30 A.M., I got a call from my brother, Fred, in California. Rob's girlfriend in Maine had been called by a friend who had gone over and found Rob dead. Rob had shot himself in the chest with a shotgun that he'd gotten at somebody's yard sale. It had happened at the same time that I had had that horrible pain. The whole thing was pretty incredible to me, especially after not being connected with Rob. We hadn't talked to each other in three years, and to have that experience—

About three months later, I had an amazing dream. The dream was of a family scene at a big table. My dad was there. People were milling around in the background. My brother, Rob, was sitting at the table. And then my mother came in from the side, from behind him, and put her arms around him and held him, hugged him. I woke up crying. It was such a beautiful image. I do take comfort in thinking of them being together.

If I would make time to be still more often, to have more still time in my life, I probably would be able to connect more with my mother and Rob. I feel like I get so wrapped up in taking care of everybody and everything that I don't allow myself enough time to sit and let myself feel their presence more. I am aware of them. I had a near-horrible accident a few years ago. I was spinning out on black ice on Route 2. At moments like that, I feel as if I have someone watching after me and taking care. You know, I feel like there's a protection there. The sense of having someone watching me is new since my mother died. I don't know what it is or how we do it, but I feel it's there.

Archer Mayor

Archer Mayor is a successful author of mystery books as well as an emergency medical technician, volunteer firefighter, and community leader. His experiences in all of those professions have provided him with a much more extensive knowledge of death than most people have. He took time out of his many commitments to visit me and share his thoughts and observations about the moment of death.

I've been doing EMS work for well over ten years, and in that time, I've probably, just in terms of rescue calls, done something in the nature of nine hundred calls. Most of those don't involve death, but quite a few have, including one just forty-eight hours ago.

Death is always nearby. It's something whose proximity doesn't distress me in the slightest. I'm comfortable with it. I'm comfortable with my interactions with it and with what I can do with it. Obviously, if I can stave death off, I'll try my damnedest to do that. And I've been successful in a number of cases. That's gratifying when you can apply your skill and your judgment to a terminal situation and turn it around. Now there's a sliding scale on that success. Clinicians will say, "That was a save" when someone is alive but he's not conscious; he's in a coma and he'll die a week later, for example. That's a save? To me, a save is when I get a postcard from the person, saying, "I'm back in my garden. Thank you very much." That's a save. Nothing else is.

A lot of the people on whom I conduct CPR really should just be left alone. But that's not my job. When I'm called on, I have certain obligations. Taking care of the elderly is much easier along those lines because they've lived full lives. When you walk into their living rooms, bedrooms, homes, trailers, you can kind of assess, just by looking at them, whether they want to fight or not. There is a sense of vitality demonstrating a will to live or a will to die. Oftentimes I'll walk in and I'll see such a scene of peace and tranquility in a dying person's face. It's different with young people. I was on a call when a three-year-old child had his chest torn open by a wolf hybrid. Now that was a case in which I did everything I could.

When we got to the hospital, the nurses and doctors did what they could, but basically that wolf had known what it was doing. The nurses were crying and the doc was grim faced and concerned, both for the nurses and for obviously everyone else involved in the process. I looked at myself and I thought, I'm not feeling anything here. I'm not feeling numbness either. I'm just feeling, Did I do everything I could do? And the answer was, Yeah, I did everything I could do.

Then I thought, What else do I feel? I feel angry. Why do I feel angry? I feel angry because some bonehead guy had to breed wolf hybrids because dogs weren't enough so he had to make some sort of monster whose instincts are of course to look at small children as meat. Why am I angry? I'm angry because the next-door neighbor who was taking care of these kids didn't have a fence around her yard, didn't have any alarm bells going off that her neighbor was breeding wolf hybrids. Because the wolf that tore up the child was a bitch who had just given birth to a whole litter, and that's of course what attracted the kid. Well, come on, you know. Where are the brains here? So perhaps I found an emotional outlet in anger at the people who were involved in this utterly senseless death. It was such a waste. This was a young child who had his whole life ahead of him. He wasn't in any position to decide that this was a good time to die.

I was holding him when he died. It's funny. I've held a lot of people when they've died, and I have read and heard reflections about the soul leaving or about a sense of passage. I have to be perfectly honest: I've never, ever experienced that in any way, shape, or form. Young, old, violent, natural, drug-induced, you name it—regardless of the cause of death, age, background, or sex of the individual, I've never, ever experienced any sign of anything other than someone just dying. And that is usually expressed, if you can hear it at all, with a final breath. Their eyes don't suddenly go wider. They don't peacefully look as if they've gone to sleep. They just stop living. Their eyes generally are at half-mast. They don't close. They don't open.

The person looks dead. He turns white, quite quickly. He becomes almost heavier, in a funny kind of way. What I'm always reminded of when I'm with my dead patients is how much fluid our bodies hold, that we are, in fact, mostly liquid. That element comes most to mind just as they die. It's extraordinary. Everything is utterly limp. There is nothing in there that's alive, which is extraordinary because I've dealt with a lot of unconscious people also. And the residual energy that keeps that body pink and resistant is not there when that person's dead.

I would imagine the life force dissipates, much as hot water turning cold dissipates its heat into the air. I would imagine that energy, electrical and otherwise, dissipates. But I've never seen it. And I don't know if it's there to be seen. I would imagine what happens to it is much the same thing that happens with heat coming off cooling water. It just goes into the atmosphere and is used in other ways. So I supposed the air we breathe is filled with dead people's energies. Well, that might be a hopeful way of looking at it. I've never really gone that far, to be honest.

In dealing with death, year in and year out, sometimes in quite traumatic settings, you've got to park your feelings somewhere, you have to park the emotional reality that you're dealing with dying human beings. If you don't have that awareness, you're a cold-hearted bastard. If you feel too much emotion, you can't do your job. So you've got to do something with the feelings. Parking is what we in EMS call it. You put your emotions in a cubbyhole. You put them in a closet. You put them behind a door somewhere.

We know, those of us who think about this, we know that what is parked will sometimes spontaneously become unparked. You may be in a boat in the middle of a lake, fishing. Pleasant, wonderful summer day, and you burst into tears. Curiously, the stimulating events that cause unparking aren't necessarily what you would expect:

machine guns flying loose, decapitated babies, and all that. Some-times it can be something incredibly minor like a car crash in which no one's injured. All of a sudden you'll see one person on the rescue squad has just lost it. He just can't cope. And you say, "Get that guy some help," because things have become unparked. The emotions have broken loose.

If you want to use a maritime metaphor, you strap that stuff down on deck and occasionally, in a tempest-tossed world, it breaks loose, and then you get loose cargo or a loose cannon flying around that will tear you up unless someone helps you lash it back down or deal with it somehow or other.

I think it's a shame in a way that we look at grief as having to be "dealt with." I have no problem with grieving twenty years later. I think that's fine. But we are structured in a technological fashion to "deal with" things. Got a problem? Deal with it. Got a loss of a loved one? Deal with it. You have assigned to you one year of mourning after a loss. After that, you can get remarried after a divorce or have another child—whatever.

People are fairly impatient and a little bit testy with grief. They'll give you free casseroles for the first week. They'll say, "How're you doing?" for the next month. After that, you'd better have dealt with it. They will tell you that it will take a year, but no one's even going to stick around that long. I think that's nonsense. I think it's proba-bly healthy if you get on with life, yet the loss may in fact make you richer than you were before. You may all of a sudden look at life in a whole different and better way. It may mean more to you, now that you've suffered this loss. So why would you want to "deal with" that, parking it away? You don't want to park it away; it's enriching you.

EMT work has made me more thoughtful, more empathetic, more patient. I used to be able to spot an asshole from three miles away. Now I'm a little hard-pressed to identify an asshole anywhere. Because I guess I can always kind of see a little bit of where they're coming from and what they're all about. Perhaps my being death's constant visitor has something to do with my being able to cut peo-ple—and myself—some slack, with my being able to be a little less judgmental.

We come, we go. We die old, we die young. We die because we

deserved it in that we lived hellacious lives of drug and alcohol abuse, or we never knew what hit us, but we're dead anyhow. So who am I to wander around judging people at random just because I'm having a bad hair day or *any* kind of hair day? I don't know for sure if that's just a sign of aging or whether that's my exposure to death.

So I've come to take death in stride, pretty much like I take the weather and a lot of other things in stride. As an EMT, the one thing that will keep me up at night will be if I screwed up, if I could have done something that I somehow spaced out because it was too wild a scene or I forgot to do it or something like that.

I have seen so much of death in familial environments, where people are weeping and crying and you are looking up from your job, which is trying to salvage this human being, and you can see the faces and the eyes, and you can hear the tension and the wonder and the denial in the voices. You can also feel them putting everything onto you: "Save my beloved. You're here. We called you, and you came, and now you're working wonderfully well and wonderful things will result." And I'm saying "This person's dead, or is just about to die, and there's no way I'm going to be able to reverse that." That happens fairly frequently. That's not a problem for me. I've chosen to put myself in this place. If I found it too tough, I'd get out of it.

Each time someone dies, death is basically the same, funny enough. It really is. It really is. Despite all its various contexts. It's very odd that way. Death is fascinating, in fact, and part of that may be due to the fact that life goes on instantly thereafter.

I don't think a whole lot about my own mortality. Maybe I don't think a whole lot about it because I see how death whacks people right out of the blue. Death will hit you upside the head whenever it feels like it. You can walk on water. You can eat tofu. You could drink yourself silly every night. I don't care what the hell you do to either speed it up or stave it off, it will grab you when it goddamn well feels like it. So I don't think about it. Because I know I may get in my car and may not even live to the end of the block after I leave my house. On the other hand, I may live to be ninety-two, like my father. Beats the hell out of me. So I'm not going to worry about it.

Once, when I was a teenager, I remember stepping into a room and all of a sudden being filled with absolute fear of dying, but not because of anything that was happening in the room. It was just the understanding that I might die, for whatever reason at whatever point, that I would eventually die, sooner or later. The fear went away in the flash of an eyelid, and that was the last time I ever felt it. I never tried to figure out why, but I couldn't. It just happened. Lots of things do.

Margaret Robinson

College administrator Margaret Robinson was helped through the difficulty of losing her husband by a supportive employer, by grown children who pitched in and assisted her with difficult tasks, and, most importantly, by a dying and loving husband who made key decisions about his own death process. Hers is a story of courage marked by a willingness to make personal decisions to honor her dying husband's final wishes.

My husband, Mike, essentially had heart failure. We had known for some years that he had a bad valve and it was getting worse—it was narrowing more and more—but he didn't want any invasive measures. He didn't want surgery or anything of the sort. Some time in January, he had a silent heart attack, of which he wasn't aware. But that, coupled with the bad valve, did enough damage to give him only about a 20 percent pumping capacity in his heart. Of course, that produced all sorts of bad symptoms, not so much with respect to pain—he never complained about pain—but with respect to breathing difficulties and the panic attacks that come when the brain isn't getting enough oxygen. It was something he really had trouble describing. He could only describe it as the most awful feeling in the world, almost like the deepest of depressions where it feels like the bottom is falling out of everything. He found his condition almost intolerable. I think he could have put up with the rest, with the pain.

This situation extended only for about two weeks total. I took him to the hospital. He was getting worse, and he stayed there for two days. Mike's own doctor was on vacation when Mike checked into the hospital, so he never saw Mike again. Mike was a month short of ninety-two. Mike just hooted and said, "Even if I survive an operation, what's the rest of my life going to be like? It will take me probably a year to recover, at which time I'll die of some other cause." Mike felt he had had a very good, rich, full, long life, and he was not going to prolong it artificially. The medications the doctors gave him weren't doing much, and the hospital said fine, Mike could take those same drugs at home. So I took him home and received a leave of absence from my job. I brought my computer home and did what I could from home whenever I had time. I was in contact with my office, but they told me just to take my time, to do whatever was needed at home.

At that point, Mike started sort of casting around for the means to speed up death. When he came home from the hospital, I think he still hoped that simply being home again would help him recover, to at least get back to living at a certain plateau. But after a week he realized that he was getting weaker, not stronger.

For a few days, he could still manage to walk down the hallway and back, to the bedroom and the bathroom. Then gradually, even that became more and more difficult. We finally rented a wheelchair for him. He hated the whole idea. He realized that there was no real medical help forthcoming. All he could look forward to were a few simple things, such as a visit by his own doctor when he came back from vacation.

We'd been given a date for an office visit with his doctor, but it became quite clear to me that I could not get Mike back to the hospital for that, so I requested that his doctor make a house call. Oooh. Impossible. It would be at least ten days to two weeks before the doctor could come. Mike's doctor offered to send his physician's assistant, a woman whom we'd seen before. So she came and she spent, oh, maybe forty minutes with Mike. She discussed his case honestly with him but made it quite clear that they weren't prepared to help him to die. They could only continue giving Mike his medication, which really wasn't doing anything. I thought Mike had reached a point where he might be eligible for Hospice. When I had checked Mike out of the hospital, I, point blank, asked the doctor who had been seeing him in the hospital what the expectations were. What should I prepare for? He said, "It could be tomorrow. It could be three weeks. It could be two months. It could be six months. We just don't know. Just be prepared; it could happen very quickly."

To me, then, it was clear that this was the final interval in Mike's life. I thought, Maybe I can get him switched to Hospice and see if we can make him more comfortable. Mike was privy to this plan. So that's what we did. Hospice people started coming in. It was really one of the Hospice nurses who pointed out that Mike had a choice, if he wished to take it. The nurse said Mike could simply discontinue the medication, food, and fluids, which was already in our directives, for both of us, in our wills. Mike said, "That's exactly what I'm going to do." So we talked about it. Of course Mike asked me how I felt about it. And since I knew how much he was afraid of becoming totally incapacitated and ending up full of tubes and needles in the hospital for an indefinite period, I could not in good conscience say, "No, I'm sorry. I don't want you to do that." I couldn't. I was grateful that I didn't have to make the decision for him, though. He was capable of deciding, This is what I want. There was no doubt in anyone's mind. Mike didn't ask me to participate; he just wanted to know if it was all right with me. It was a good thing that we had talked about it often enough previously so that I knew what was really important to him.

Mike stopped eating and drinking the next day, all at the same time. The Hospice nurses gave him low-grade morphine, which eased the breathing and the anxiety attacks tremendously without knocking him out. In the beginning, Mike used morphine several times a day. Then the nurses had to increase the dosage. Mike was conscious for all but the last twenty-four hours, although not able to speak. He could react, yes, but he couldn't speak. He was too dehydrated and too weak. On Saturday, which was actually the fourth day since he had begun, the nurses said, "It probably will be a few more hours, but we don't think it will be much longer." Well, it was another twenty-four hours. Somehow, Mike still had tremendous resources even though he had lost a lot of weight. He was down to about one hundred and twenty-five pounds. We didn't know where that energy was coming from. He hadn't been ill except for his narrowing valve, which they knew about, and his eyesight. He had macular degeneration and could no longer read. But other than that, he had been very lucky. We all had been very lucky.

I really was a little uneasy about what was happening. I had never been exposed to death in any intimate way. All three children came to visit, one from the West Coast. The other two live in the East. I wasn't sure how our children would deal with it. But I needn't have worried. They pitched in immediately. Each one picked an area they thought they could handle best. Leslie made herself responsible for the phone and answering the door and dealing with all the things she didn't want us to have to deal with. Patrick, our son, dealt with things like the catheter changing and all that sort of thing. Our middle daughter, who's married and has children, and I took over the nursing duties in between the nurses' visits. He knew we were there. One of us was with him the whole time and sometimes two or three of us. Someone was always sitting there holding his hand. And he could respond by giving a squeeze. We would turn Mike and do whatever we could for him or sit with him, talk to him. We talked gently about people and things with which we thought he might be concerned in this passage, such as his brother, who had died before him, and his son, who had committed suicide ten years earlier.

In the first of those five days, he was really quite weak and didn't speak a lot. But he could understand us and he could articulate. We talked about some of his family, about the past, and about things that he wished he had done, a few unresolved things, but nothing major, really. He kept saying he was glad to have had the life he had, that he felt very grateful for it, and how full it had been. He said he was grateful for his family and for the people around him. He was very grateful for the nurses, too, the Hospice people. He joked with them. The aide came to help, and he would tease her. He didn't lose his sense of humor till the very end, when he went into the coma. It was quite amazing, too, which again helped us because he had many opportunities along the way to change his mind about what he had chosen to do, and he didn't. It didn't occur to him; he was happy to be going.

Several other people came to see him in the last few days, including friends of ours from California. When they were leaving, Mike grabbed Bob's hand and held onto it for a while and said, "Robert, I'm glad to see you." Mike's niece, his favorite niece, came from New York to help, too. She had come once before, when Mike was first home from the hospital, and had stayed for two or three days. She stayed for a couple of days again during the last week. When the children all arrived, she left again. He liked having her around.

In the final days, there wasn't anything that the outside world did that was helpful for Mike. He was done with that part of life, that aspect of it—the outside. He was drawing in and concentrating on his immediate situation. The neighbors of course were very helpful. Most of them came and brought food and asked if they could help. A friend who lived across the street was a nurse, so she came by early on when he first came home from the hospital. She gave me lots of good information and advice and tips on how to physically handle things. Another friend from down the street became a Hospice volunteer, even though it was only for a week or two. She came several times so that I could run out for half an hour and do something.

Those last five days were possible because I think Mike knew we two were on a pretty firm foundation. Nobody had given us a chance, when we married, for the marriage to survive more than a few years. He was fifty-five and I was twenty-six. He was fifty-three when we met. We ourselves didn't know how long it would last, but we thought it was worth trying. But it never occurred to either of us to change it, once we started. Yes, I think he felt secure enough, and loved enough, to choose this final path. As far as I could tell, he was comfortable doing what he did, and peaceful. As difficult as it was, we were glad and proud to help him do it.

The really difficult part for us was the Cheyne-Stokes breathing that sets in after a while. It went on for a long, long time—two and a half days, maybe. He would stop breathing for sometimes a couple of minutes at a time and we would think, This is it, and then he'd start again. But then when he went into a coma during his last twenty-four hours, that rough breathing stopped. He started to breathe almost normally. But then at the very end, the last hour or two, Cheyne-Stokes started again. Very strange. He didn't move *at all* from his position. We did turn him a couple of times because he was beginning to develop some sores, and the nurses said, "If you can, just turn him gently," and we did. But he was really unresponsive at that point, both physically and mentally. Yet I didn't have the feeling that it was painful for him or that he was really bothered by it. He seemed peaceful, in spite of that.

The best we could do was keep telling him it was all right to let go. All of us told him. I wasn't always there when the children were alone with him, but I know our son told him how proud he was to be his son, which was great, because you know it was difficult for Patrick some of the time having a father so much older than the other kids' fathers. My husband was something like sixty-one when Patrick was born. Since Mike was retired at the time, he was often pressed into service to drive sports teams around and all that sort of thing. He was always the one on whom they could rely.

But because Mike was always so much younger than his age, it really didn't make a difference. He and Patrick could still play tennis together and ski together and do everything else. Patrick kept saying to his father, "Gee, I hope when I get to be your age I can look back and say 'I've done this, that, and that.' It will be great." Patrick was able to say that to his father, which was wonderful for both of them.

Most of my husband's career was spent in the foreign service, but during the war, for instance, he was the first program director for AFN in London, the American Forces Network. He was one of the founders of the AFN. He was a writer all his life. He published a novel, several plays, short stories, and what have you. He was still doing that right up to the end. Mike had had a very active life and had something to show for it.

The whole stretch of watching the gradual decline and the various stages as they set in was quite profound for all of us. But the thing that helped us the most was knowing how sure Mike was that this was the way he wanted it to be. He wanted to be at home with his family and go in peace. That's what he did. That's what was happening. His advance directives stated, "No heroic measures, and, in fact, withholding food and fluids." So he really did nothing different from what he had determined to do years before. We had talked about it often in the last few years. He'd had one or two very small strokes that really didn't have any impact on him beyond a couple of weeks of weakness in an arm or leg, but each time, of course, he knew it brought him closer to his end.

The thing I'm still sort of awed by is what happened at the very end. Mike hadn't moved in twenty-four hours—hadn't moved an eyelid or a muscle or anything—but he suddenly opened his eyes for about, oh, maybe three or four seconds, but not focusing on anything. The expression on his face was not one of seeing but one of listening. You can tell when people just sort of look off to the side, you know they're trying to hear something. That was exactly what he looked like. And then it was over. That was it.

Being without food and dehydrated for five days and not having much to draw on in the first place, his face had become very sharp featured, the way faces do. And then almost immediately after his death, it started to smooth out. It was miraculous. He didn't look like the same person. It was almost like his face filled in again a little bit. He looked completely different. He looked more like himself. I'm still puzzling over that. He never regained his color. It had already changed, days before. It was the typical waxy sheen, and that didn't change, but the features did become more like the way he used to look. I have puzzled over both these things—the distinct listening quality of that one moment when he opened his eyes again and the way his face changed. The Hospice nurses said sometimes people see people from their past. He might have. Maybe he saw his brother. He was very attached to his older brother, who had died about seven or eight years earlier. Or maybe he saw his mother. Whatever it was, it was something he really didn't want to miss. I could tell that.

At the moment of death, his presence changed quickly. Then I had the feeling that it was more or less a shell that was there, it was just his body going through the last involuntary motions, breathing still. Those last few seconds, though, when he opened his eyes and cocked his ears, he was there again. But then, very pronouncedly, he was not there as soon as it was over.

Mike had become a member of New Hampshire's Cremation Society. The Hospice nurse had called, and she came within an hour, an hour and a half of Mike's death, and I let the children deal with that part. That was one thing I couldn't do. Maybe that was cowardly, but the nurse and I had gotten him ready before, put his pajamas on, combed his hair, that sort of thing. That I could do, but I couldn't be there when they took him away. That was too much.

I stayed home for about a week after he died and took care of a lot of legal stuff and paperwork and notifying. I found I really couldn't concentrate on anything for any length of time. I was sitting most of the time just staring out of the window. I finally said, "This is no good for anybody," so I went back to work. I felt in limbo, I wasn't even there. I couldn't seem to gather myself together enough to move forward, move out of it. I've had trouble sleeping ever since. Hopefully, some day that will abate. The only thing I have to be distressed about is the loss, the absence. He isn't fully absent, though. It's hard to describe, but it's as though he's never far away and sort of still knows what's going on to some extent. There's a consciousness in that presence, not an interactive one, but it's there in some ways; it's not that far away. It's fine. It's certainly not uncomfortable. It's something I'm glad to have.

Mike was a remarkable man. He was quite amazing. He never, never liked to make waves for himself. In fact, he would have been absolutely astonished at so many people even taking notice of his passing. He was surprisingly humble. He had lived a fairly quiet life the last few years because he was really confined to quarters here until I came home. People would come to see us occasionally. We'd have a few friends over for dinner, but so many of the people in his generation had died off. There really weren't any left. His overriding interest in life was people. He was very outgoing, very gregarious, and had a wonderful gift of drawing people out. He could talk to anybody and get them to respond. Any age. Really quite remarkable. I thought it absolutely fabulous that Mike could reach a point where he could say, "Well, this is it, and it's been great, but now it's time to go on." Most people I have known in a similar situation before were determined to hang on, literally, for dear life.

We had bought a grave plot in a local cemetery because the children really wanted one spot to go to where there is a marker. Mike wanted just a plain, flat marker with his name and the dates, and that was it. That's exactly what he got.

When the children and I were in Nantucket at the same time, we went out very early one morning and scattered most of his ashes in his favorite places on the island; one place was a very isolated pond on the moors. That was another amazing experience. It was about 7:00 in the morning, an overcast day. It was the week of the tail end of Hurricane Bonnie, the last week in August. We walked along the edge of the pond to get away from the access road. Just as we started walking along and Patrick started scattering the ashes, the sun broke through the clouds and these huge swaths of light came down—you know, the diffused light that you get—and a big flock of white birds settled on the lake. We looked at each other; we had shivers going up and down our spines.

So, yes, so he's in the local cemetery and in Nantucket, in two places—one beach and one pond—and right here in the house, too. The poor man is in four different places. I am totally comfortable having him here. I'd go in and talk to him when his ashes were still in the house. We had him cremated in February, and we didn't spread his ashes anywhere until summer. I had him here in the house for quite a while—in fact, until two days ago. I was working outside two days ago and I picked a spot that Mike had always said was a place where he wanted to do something useful—he wanted his ashes to feed some flowers or bushes. He considered that. So I said, "Mike, you're going to get your wish." That was one of his favorite flowerbeds, and it's where the dog is scattered. He and the dog were very attached to each other. We had her for fifteen years, and she died a few years ago. He didn't want another dog. He didn't want to get attached again to an animal that way, especially one that would outlive him. So the dog had been cremated and scattered on the lawn down below where she had always hung around. She had had the same kind of life as Mike, a very good life, sick for three days, at age fifteen. But they had walked together every day. He had fed her. She used to sit right beside him, and everywhere he went, she went. When he was at the typewriter, she would be in there. When he was in the living room, she'd be there, too. She would not be anywhere but where he was. Maybe it was the dog that he was listening to in that final moment.

I'm convinced there is something more to this existence but that we know nothing about it. It isn't the usual "white light at the end of the tunnel," I am sure. I talked to my brother in Germany who had a bypass a year and a half ago and who actually died during the operation and had to be revived, a fact that his doctors didn't tell him until well afterward. I asked my brother what it was like and if he had any recollection if he had experienced anything unusual. He said, "Nothing. Absolutely nothing."

But the way Mike died was completely for the rest of us. I think it's something the children will not forget, either. It was such a lesson in courage and dignity—and love—for all of us. These are things about a person you can't know when you marry them. Even after more than thirty or forty years, until it happens, you don't know what they will decide and how they're going to react. Whenever we'd talked about it in the past, he would ask me if there was anything that I could think of, when the time came, to help him die. I told him I couldn't, and even if I could, I didn't think I *could* assist him like that. I don't think I could have, even if I had known what to do. I assisted him, in a way, just by agreeing, but that's as far as I could have gone, actively.

Mike is still with me. It is not just here that I feel his presence. It's wherever I go. But it's not oppressive, it's not uncomfortable, it's not disapproving or approving. It's just there. So it's very much like the kind of companionship we had these last few years. There weren't a whole lot of things left that we could do together that required physical effort, so most of our relationship was just sitting here in the evenings and having meals—just companionship—and that was fine. That's sort of what it feels like now. And as I say, I still talk to him. It's better than talking to myself.

Frances M. VanDaGriff

Frances VanDaGriff, director of The Homestead, an elder-care residence home, was with her close friend, Dona, throughout the months of Dona's death from cancer. Frances, who had grown up in a culture and family that kept children buffered from death, ended up in a profession that taught her to handle death openly. Her experiences have enabled her to understand and celebrate people's lives as they are dying and to cherish their memories after they are gone.

My mother died when I was three. My grandfather committed suicide when I was probably one and a half. And I was never allowed to go to a funeral. Where I lived, in Oklahoma, people just seemed to disappear. I didn't know anything about death until I moved to Vermont. I had never been to a funeral, literally. I came to New England as a young mother, in my thirties. I had still never attended a funeral. I had attended a memorial service, you know, no body, no nothing. Then I got a job at The Homestead. The Homestead is right next door to a funeral home. And as residents started to die, which they do here, there would be visiting hours in the funeral home. The first body I ever saw was at visiting hours. That was the first funeral I had been to. I was in my mid-thirties at least. I saw the common sense of it; people didn't simply disappear. Friends were allowed to stand up and talk and remember things. I got used to that part of it. I liked the closure.

I got the job at The Homestead by living next door. I was teaching preschool. The lady who ran The Homestead at that time came over and asked if I would be willing to work at the desk on the weekends and take care of residents. They're very independent; it's a level-three facility. I needed the Christmas money, so I said yes. And then The Homestead needed a weekend cook, and I did that for a while. And then I became the assistant director, and then I became the director. That's when I started learning about death, about the other side of death—not the disappearance kind.

Then my friend Dona got oral cancer. We went through a whole bunch of denial, as friends. Our kids were the same ages. We had found ourselves to be kindred spirits. We were both adult children of alcoholics. She had never had anybody just up and say, "Well, my parents were alcoholics." They had kept it in the background. And so I said, "Oh, by the way, I have a real compulsive personality because I'm an adult child of alcoholics. My humor and all my gregariousness is a cover so people won't get real close." And she said, "Oh really?" So after that, we were fine. We studied reincarnation together, on our own, as friends. We studied several religions. Adult children of alcoholics don't do anything without a plan. They always have to be prepared for anything that's going to shock them. I have an emergency kit in my car. You never know. That was the way we did things. We prepared for her cancer in that fashion. We read *Many Lives, Many Masters,* by Leavenson. We read many eclectic books. We started going to the health food store because someone said, "Macrobiotics—the only way." Then she started gargling with peroxide and snorting it up her nose because she had heard that cancer needs air, and hydrogen peroxide takes away air. She tried that, and of course it burned out her sinuses something fierce.

She had the option of having her soft palette removed. But she was vain, and she said, "The cancer is probably going to kill me anyway, and I'm not going to go around with food getting stuck in the roof of my mouth and going God knows where." She had the cancer removed, but she didn't have any bone removed. We did this for six years, and during that time, there would be times when she would go into denial. "I don't have cancer." "I'm going to beat this thing." I never knew which Dona I was going to see each morning. I had to wait until she opened her mouth to find out where we were going with our thoughts. That was perhaps the hardest part, because she would flip and flop, back and forth. "I'm just going to give in and die and do it gracefully." The next day: "No, I'm going to go here and there and do this. We're going to fight this thing." I felt like I was on the wildest stagecoach ride I've ever been on.

Dona and I did a lot of walking, a lot of talking. And finally, I started amassing extra hours at The Homestead. I was assistant director then. I started working every overtime hour they had, all the extra shifts, and amassing those to use for comp time. I asked my boss. I said, "Please, can I amass these hours so that when it comes time that Dona needs a caregiver, I can be part of that team?" She said, "No problem."

I would call Dona and she wouldn't answer. I finally would go out on the weekend and she would act hurt and angry that I hadn't been there. I finally told Angie, Dona's daughter, "I called her all week long but she's always out." And Angie said, "No, the cancer is in her ear. She can't hear now." So there had been a turn. Dona thought I was ignoring her. I took her on a last trip to Maine. We used to love to go to Maine together. We stayed at the beach. It was in the early spring. She was doing it more for me than for herself. Also there were times she needed to get away from her family. She would get angry with them because they would try to take care of her. She was a nurse. Toward the end, she had gotten her nursing degree—a last-minute thing. Her family didn't meet her standards of caregivers sometimes, so she'd get very miffed with them. She told me I was a lousy caregiver, too. And I said, "Just shut up and roll over." We would laugh.

We went to the beach the first couple of days we were there. When we were going to the beach, Dona would walk out across the parking lot, just oblivious to cars. I thought, "Well, she's just going to die right here. I'm not going to have to worry about the last rites." People would honk and curse at her, and she'd smile and give them the thumbs up. That was her favorite thing, the thumbs-up thing. I would just shrug my shoulders and push her along.

Toward the end of her life, she tried taking all her pills at once. She took ninety morphine pills and twenty Percocet at home. Her daughter called me and said, "I think Mom's taken all her pills." I went over there, and we began doing the deathwatch with her, waiting for her to go. But she didn't die. She woke up with a look on her face like, "Oh damn it. It didn't work." She looked ticked off.

As people die or go into their final death process, they might choose you as the friend they want to be there. They might not want their cousin, someone who might want to be too close, in the circle. For a dying person, the circle of acceptable people gets smaller and smaller. Dying people don't suffer fools gladly. They pick premium people, and toward the end there might be only four or five whom they allow in. We had about six, and they were all on the bed that day, along with a German shepherd and a cat with worms. Dona would minister to us like Mother Teresa or something. She was drunker than a skunk from the pills. It was hysterical. We spent the whole day with her, about half of it laughing and the rest of it crying. And then she began to see people outside the window. There were "men" outside the window, waiting for her. It was in her mind. We kept telling her, "It's probably not angels. It's the FBI. Have you paid your taxes?" And, oh, she thought that was hysterical. She still had a sense of humor. It very well could have been some messengers. We don't know that side yet. We stayed with her the whole time. We made it through. Drank a lot of coffee. Laughed a lot. Oh, she was funny.

Dona's reason for taking the pills had been that she didn't want to see any more cancer doctors. She said, "I got in there, and I paid them money just to have them tell me I'm dying and I'm doing a good job of it? That's for the birds. They don't need to see me." But the doctors wouldn't give her the pain medication unless she came into the office. I said to her husband, "Let's take her into the health center." By now, the cancer had grown through her right cheekbone. She had a big sore and a bulging pink mass coming out under her eye. She was disfigured, and she was very vain. She knew everybody in town.

I called one of the local doctors and explained what was going on. He said, "You come in and get the pills. She doesn't have to come in here. She's dying. You're right." He had compassion. But he said, "I have to meet her once." So I told Dona, "We can get this thing going. Do you want to go in or do you want him to come here?" She said, "No, I'll go in." She was still drunk from her overdose. And so we went in and he figured out what she had taken and he said, "If you can beat that, I wouldn't be at all surprised what you can beat." He just sat there and laughed with her.

After that, I would go in and get the prescriptions, and she never had to see another doctor. She could just stay home. We borrowed a wheelchair from The Homestead. We borrowed a commode, too. After that, Dona pretty much stayed in bed. It got to where her family would come home and find that she had gotten up on a chair and painted a blue line around the edges of the ceiling, just because it seemed like a good idea to do. Of course, her balance was totally off and they were very worried about leaving her alone. So I started using my amassed days. I think I did Tuesdays and Thursdays as her caregiver. She said she didn't want any strangers coming in. She didn't want this person, that person, all these other people. She had a list of who she didn't want in. I said, "Okay, that's fine. I'll make sure they don't come. How about Hospice, the volunteers?" She said, "Nope. No way. Kids can do it. You can do it. We'll be fine." I said, "All right." And she told me how to do oral care. That was a big problem. She used to brush her teeth eight times a day. She said, "I want my mouth clean." I looked up her durable power of attorney for health, and it said, "No heroics but plenty of oral care." Oh, it's a grungy thing to do, but we made it through.

Dona found out how expensive morphine was, and she said, "Well, why don't we try an alternative drug?" There was a drug they used for addicts who were coming down. It's not morphine, and it's very inexpensive. She said, "I'd like to try that." She called the doctor and he said, "Fine, it's much cheaper." That cut her costs in half for about two months. So she was still in control.

Dona's kids wanted a life. They were something like ten, fourteen, and sixteen or eighteen, around that age. They didn't want to sit with their mother all the time. They would go out on the patio and talk to friends, and she would do something crazy the second they were gone. I said, "Can we bring the Hospice people in?" We had one come over, and Dona was very nice to her. But then she said, "No. No. I don't want any more Hospice."

I said, "I think your kids and husband need Hospice. Can we do it for them? I think they need it." It was the first time I was able to manipulate her. Dona said, "What if I don't like these people?" And I said, "Then pretend to be asleep." I said, "They'll work quietly around you and leave. Just pretend to be asleep if they annoy you." She was very private, so okay, that was the plan. Well, it worked a little too well because one time I was in there and we were watching TV and she wanted me to see—oh, it was some friendly little neighborhood show that was like a soap opera. I was very bored with it, and I was sewing. She just kept flicking the channels, channel surfing. I hate that. She knows it. And so I turned to talk to her and she shut her eyes and pretended to be asleep. She was giving me the message: "You can take your caregiving and take it out the door!"

We went through that for a while. Weeks. Weeks. Weeks. From spring till July we had pretty much round-the-clock caregivers. She finally started slipping into longer and longer sleep spells. She had a voracious appetite that couldn't be satisfied. I sometimes find that with these folks as they get near death. I wonder if they're feeding the cancer. At some point in the dying process, it seems like we have a lot of big eaters and then it quiets down. I don't know why. It's just something I've noticed.

Dona had a ravenous appetite for ice cream. We'd make her coddled eggs—all soft food. In the meantime, she had made a quilt for each child. She had amassed a freezer full of casseroles and breads for the family, for when she was gone, so that they could use those during their grief. She had taken and copied her recipes twice for the girls, so that they each had a recipe book. She had made a teddy—a little frilly teddy—for the youngest girl, so that she would have something later on. The child wasn't ready for it yet. But Dona knew she'd want something fancy some day. And the kids, in the meantime, had—during the period when Dona was a little bit better in the winter—done a special celebration for her. I think it was their parents' anniversary. The evening came complete with catered food from a fancy restaurant and the right songs. It was just exotic. The oldest daughter set it up, and then she farmed out the younger two kids and herself. There was this give and take, always, back and forth. It was very nice.

The week before Dona died, it was a hot July day, and there was a window at the head of Dona's bed, and everybody was on the bed all the time. I was reading Dona's notebook, which was filled with all sorts of spiritual quotes about getting over cancer and life hereafter, quotes that she had amassed during the past six years. The Hospice nurse was bathing her, and the sun was coming in. It could have been a scene from a movie, it really could have. The pace of everything was so very slow. I'm fast. I do everything quickly. But the nurse was washing between Dona's fingers. She moved her ring up a little and washed under it and moved it down and washed. She washed the curl in Dona's ear and gave her a shampoo and did under her nails, and I thought, Good heavens. And then it dawned on me that this might be her last bath. The nurse was doing it almost like a religious rite. Inch by inch, she was bathing Dona, and I was paying attention to all of it. And then the nurse asked me to read aloud. I thought, Eh? And it dawned on me that the nurse was taking care of me. That's when I kind of fell apart. All along, I had thought that I didn't need attention! I'm quite self-sufficient. I need no one. I've learned to take care of myself, and here was this nurse is taking care of me. And I thought, Oh, God.

Dona died later that week, and I was with her for the last forty-eight hours. The same people who had been there at the suicide scene were there again. And she managed to do things up. She managed to say good-bye to each person. Her children and her husband and her mother and father were there. Her sister came. I was there. Some people had a tendency to get out of the room because there was a horrible smell. It was a rotten-meat smell. Dona had gone into a coma and was starting to do the Cheyne-Stokes breathing, which reminds you of a bellows. And then the breath gets slower and shallower. For a while, her breathing was just like a steam engine, and all that smell was coming out into the room. We had six people in there. We were ready to faint from the smell. I was crocheting in the corner, and I just stayed there. Everybody else came and went as they could. I sat by a window.

That evening, she was still Cheyne-Stokes breathing, and we were giving her morphine suppositories. The oldest daughter and I did it. I did most of the suppositories because the daughter really didn't feel comfortable doing it. At this point, Dona's fingers were blue and her toes were blue. The suppositories provided a little comic relief. When I was doing them, I thought, "No, no, she's still not comfortable. I can tell," even though it was me that was not comfortable, not her. When I did the last suppository, I thought, Boy, that went in easily. Very, very easily. It was only 11:30 or 12:00. I called the health center and I said, "We're out of morphine suppositories. It's the weekend and the middle of the night and she's dying." Some sweet little nurse or nurse practitioner or doctor—somebody answered—and she said, "Well, I'll tell you what. Come on down. I'll do up some more pain needles for you. Have you ever given a shot?" I said, "No." She said, "Well, I'll give you a fast lesson."

So I drove all the way in. The woman taught me how to give injections on a Styrofoam cup and then on a piece of fruit. Then she prepared about four needles. She said, "If you're telling me the truth of your observations and she's blue, you may not need any of these." She gave me the needles. I thought, Boy, everybody in town knows me pretty much because I run The Homestead, but she's certainly trusting. I left. I don't even know if she gave me morphine. She may have given me saline solution. She just kind of handed the needles to me, and I left and got back to Dona's, and the kids came home and Dona proceeded to slip on away.

My doctor friend at the health center had told me all the things to watch for. He said, "If she has a bowel obstruction, you call me and we're removing her from the house. Her family doesn't need to endure that, and she wouldn't have them do so. If you suspect an obstruction, that's one time you call me." He gave me all the rules. He gave me what to look for, and that was so helpful.

Dona's circulation was slowing down, her breathing was just from part of her lungs or maybe from just the diaphragm. Maybe a month earlier, I had given the doctor a map to her house so that when I needed to call him for the final checkout, he would be there. Oh, all these little plans. It's just like, "Oh, what dress shall I wear?"

We sat there with her. The kids finally went to a friend's house to just get away from it all. They got back about 1 A.M., and Dona died at about 1:15, after she was sure that they were home. There is a piece of dying people that stays cognizant even though they appear to be in coma. It was pretty obvious that she waited for the kids to get home, because she could have gone long before that.

We had a stethoscope—hers from nursing—and finally we listened to all the extremities and there was no heartbeat. So I made the call to the doctor, and Mark went out into the living room and was watching Mr. Bean, a British comedian, and laughing. The kids were watching Mr. Bean and laughing because we were all just in shock. It had been such a long ordeal that it was like, "Okay, this part's over. Tomorrow we'll take care of her again." I thought, "I better clean her up a little."

I found the suppository—I had put it up her vagina. It had come back out. I thought, Oh, no wonder it didn't work. Oh, I bet she's pissed at me. Oh, I'll bet I'm in trouble for this one. So I'm in there laughing, too, and cleaning her up, and thinking, Oh, Lord, I knew that was too easy.

We never did use the needles. The doctor came. We were all sitting at the dining room table making jokes, and he was checking on us. He was a young doctor but he knew that we weren't really okay. He stayed around for a while. I said, "Do you want those needles?" And he said, "Oh, yeah, yeah, yeah." I said, "Are they really morphine?" And he said, "You'll always wonder, won't you?" Then he took them away because we didn't want them left there with teenagers in a state of shock.

We held a memorial service for her at the house, and everybody told stories about her. Her favorite song was, "A Horse Named Wildfire." So we found it and we played it. Then a woman I know named Gina came to me and said, "We have a support group, a bereavement group. It would be really good if the girls came to it." And I said, "Okay, fine. I'll tell the girls they need to go to it." And Gina said, "I don't know that they have a way to get there. You've been such a part of this. Maybe you'd like to join, too." I said, "Well, I'll talk to the girls." They wouldn't go unless I went, so I said, "This is my final thing for Dona. I'll take the girls to the support group."

So we went to this bereavement group, and it was a group made up of very different types of people. And I was there with the two girls. Initially I thought I was only there for the girls, but suddenly I found I was dealing with my mother's death, my aunt's death, my grandmother's death, my father's death. I didn't talk about the others; I only spoke of Dona. It really was a very cathartic situation. Bereavement groups are marvelous. I would recommend them to anybody, even if they lost a cat. It's just very, very healthy.

I think we had met about ten times when Angela and Jessica said, "Can we have a dinner and have everybody bring the favorite food of the person who died?" And so we did. We had pizzas! Something like nine pizzas. We had Coke in the old-fashioned bottles—it had to be in the old-fashioned bottles. We had those horrible orange peanut candies that are like Styrofoam. They taste ugh. And several other odd things like chocolate gooeys. All this blaugh. But we had more fun, sharing the favorite foods of the favorite people. Then we decided that we had just had too much fun altogether. We didn't really want to break up. Gosh, that was in '93, '94. We're still meeting on a monthly basis. We've had a wedding in the group. We've seen a daughter of someone in the group get married. We've enjoyed it; we've made friends we would never have made otherwise. And they're people you might not even think you wanted to associate with. I'm sure others might have said about me, "She talks too much. Let's go the other way." But the group has been great. In addition, it has certainly served me well at The Homestead, because now that we're doing Hospice at The Homestead, I have some idea of how to support the families and the friends. I know the process. I know the signs of death. I know how to maybe shut up once in a while—though not very often!

Actually, we've had some very fun deaths at The Homestead. I don't know if it's an appropriate thing to say, but it is fun. The final hours together are where people come away feeling like they did it right for their mom or dad and that it was joyful, that they got some closures or maybe even some openings. The one thing I can do now is I can sit by somebody who is dying, and I can hug them and kiss them. Once I do it, it gives the family permission to do the same. You know, you're not going to catch death. We're always touching the dying. That's just a rule. We touch. Our caregiving team has turned out to be the staff here. They, when they're off duty, like to do the Hospice care because we fall in love with these people.

It's a heck of a lot different dealing with a resident's death than the death of someone in my family. You do become a little more professional. But you can still feel all this stuff. And that's nice. I wouldn't say I protect myself from it; I just walk in with waders and try to slop through it. I don't try to put up any walls against it, but I can step back and say, "Now, that person's being left out. We need to make sure that he is okay."

The Homestead's guestroom is a Hospice room. The first time we decided to do Hospice, a lot of folks said, "Won't it depress the residents? Won't it be depressing for those living here to have to watch people dying?" We don't bring people in here to die. But for the people who have been here for a long time, we allow them to die at home. This is their home.

We had a gentleman who had been here quite a while. His wife had been at the nursing home next door at the same time, and she had died over there. So he was still with us. He was doing fine, but he had a health problem and ended up at the hospital. It turned out that they were going to have to do a colostomy or something, and he was confused. His daughter said, "No more. Just no more. It's an indignity, and he's always been so independent." The hospital said, "You need to put him in the nursing home or take him home because we don't just wait for people to die here. These beds are for the sick." His daughter called me, just so upset, and said, "I just can't take him home." And I said, "Of course you can't. His home is here. Bring him on home." She said, "But he's dying." I said, "But he's a resident here. Bring him on home."

I announced it to the residents at breakfast. I said, "Mr. Mills is coming home to die." There was a round of applause. It was the first case where we actually brought somebody back to die, and it seemed kind of apparent. The residents had only seen people fade. When someone they know is dying here, the residents are encouraged to come in and visit. Everyone knew that Mr. Mills was in Hospice. I thought that was very nice. Quite a few of the residents came in and visited with the family. Some avoided it like the plague. But enough of them came in to do the socially correct thing because they had been through so many deaths in their own lives that they knew what to do.

We have a fellow here in Hospice right now. He had an option.

He said he wanted to go to a hospital. We said, "Okay, this is it. You've got your diagnosis. Do you want to stay here until you want to go to a hospital? Do you want to go to the nursing home, where you have all the extra oxygen and whatever you'll need?" We don't do oxygen here unless a patient is in Hospice. Prior to being in Hospice, he might have needed oxygen. It might have made him more comfortable. That's another option. We gave him all his options. He's very, very much in control of his money, and he said, "Let's write it down." So we wrote out the different costs for all of these options for him. He decided that he would much rather stay at The Homestead, so this is where he is. We just told him, "None of the rules apply to you any more. You don't have to come out to meals. You don't have to be dressed totally for meals." If a resident wants to come out in his robe and have breakfast, that's a no-no here. But not for this man.

I firmly believe in life after death. I have a firm belief that people go on to something more. Their mind and their spirit goes on to something more. I don't need to test it. I figure I'll find out when I go. I've been watching the way we can put people into that state in which they see a tunnel and lights as a result of sleep deprivation. That can be caused by a chemical we all have in our brains. The medical world is negating that experience to some extent, but I thought, Why is it there? Why do we all have it? I'm not going to second-guess that. I assume there is a plan that says maybe I don't need to know everything. I'm finally letting go of my planning—getting a little trust. Perhaps it's something I've learned from death. I don't have to plan as much. I can have more faith. I can be more comfortable. It frees me to give up total control. Dona's death taught everybody to live in the moment, to say, "I love you," now. That change has continued. Nobody in the family holds a grudge too long, and it was a real grudge-holding family. They mend their fences quickly now. We all have responded that way.

I started doing this with Dona and have done it ever since then when I've been with other dying people—I wish them a safe journey, out loud. I stroke their brow and kiss them and wish them well. After the cessation of breathing, they're still hovering. They're still hovering, I'm sure. They're in there, they're aware. I suspect that on the one hand they're heading to a neat thing, maybe—I don't know. On the other, I think my own feeling would be that if I were dying, I would be worried about the person left behind. I would be there for them, saying, "I'm booking out now. You're going to be okay. All right?"

We had a nice little Jewish lady in The Homestead. She was a very brittle diabetic. I went to her after all this study with Dona, and I said, "Mildred, if I ever come in here and find you dead, may I take your pulse? May I touch your body?" Because gentiles aren't supposed to touch a Jewish body. She said, "Oh, that's a bunch of stuff. Of course you can touch my body." And lo and behold, the caregiver who was on that night found her dead and called me up. There she was, and it was very easy to kiss her and wish her well, then, and to wish her a safe voyage and to tell her that we appreciated all she'd given us. It was easy. I still think people who have just died are here and able to hear us. They may be here forever. Maybe they're always in and out. Who knows? I have no idea. I only know that I have that opportunity to say that. Dying is a time-space thing in which people actually go someplace. They may be over there, but maybe they're still able to hear. I don't know. And maybe they're not there at all. Maybe they've turned into an electric force and they merely just sense. I don't know. It's not mine to know. But it is one last chance, while you've got the body there, to say those things.

After one of our little ladies died, the lightbulb in a lamp in my office kept being unscrewed. We decided that she was doing that. Her name was Persus. I said, "Persus is messing with the light." We have a lot of little friends around here to whom we still talk. We've kept Persus's hat out here; it's out on the wall. We've kept another lady's apron in the kitchen. We collect mementos. We've now begun to have a closure ceremony here because residents don't necessarily like to go to a funeral home or to a funeral in a church because it's too crowded. They can't hear. They're worried about whether they can get to the bathroom. So we get along just fine here. We have the ceremony here, and we get the photos of the person out. We invite a minister to do a brief religious lead-in and closure, and then we just do a celebration of the person's life as we knew it. We invite the families. They tell us the other stories. We usually tape them and give them to the family. The residents love that. The staff all comes back. We've got as many funny stories as anybody. That's nice. Something we've learned is that the ritual and the ceremony are very important.

I think another thing I've learned about death is that I wouldn't keep a child from a funeral. I maybe wouldn't take a child to a big, elaborate funeral, but I would make sure that there was an opportunity for family closure and that the child was part of it. I don't think having three or four different closures for different age groups is a bad thing. I worry about children getting lost in the shuffle.

At the local funeral home, what they do is wonderful. They give teddy bears to all the children. They have a video that talks about death. When my husband's uncle died, the local funeral home took care of the arrangements, and we went to the visiting hours. His two little granddaughters were there. I was very aware of them. They were waiting because it was an open casket. We were doing the "line thing." I was behind the two little girls. The youngest one said, "He really doesn't look like himself." And I said, "No, he doesn't have the corner of his mouth cocked up in that grin, does he?" And she said, "No. And when you pinch him, it stays standing up!" There were all these little pinch marks on his hand. She'd been pinching on Grandpa. The girls also had tucked letters into the casket. They had written their grandfather letters. They had drawn pictures for him. There were the little girls, right there. They just went from group to group of the mourners, trying to learn more. They were gleaning information because we talk our grownup talk but we wouldn't think to sit down and talk to an eight-year-old. That was interesting.

I was talking to somebody else who said, "Do you think Uncle Benny believed in God?" I said, "I really don't know, but I don't think it matters." I think we're all in for a rude shock because we have these preconceived notions. I've created my little illusion and everybody else has created theirs. Then we find out the truth. It may be better; it may be average; we may go "Oh, ho-hum." We're all going to find out at some point. But I'm sure Uncle Benny was surprised.

It's fun to give people their own little afterlife personality. An angry person may just turn into a happy person. I would hate to think that I was going to be on a cloud with a harp, though. Raugh. I can't play a note! I can't dance!

Diane D. Guerino

School health administrator Diane D. Guerino readily agreed to meet with me to share her story of the loss of her husband, Fredo, after a Hospice volunteer connected the two of us. Diane and I met in a small café by a river, where we talked for hours. Her personal story of recovery from this immense loss—a story not included in the pages that follow—involved her finally finding love again after losing her childhood sweetheart.

My husband and I met when I was a sophomore in high school and he was a junior. We were high school sweethearts. Fredo—Alfred Alfonso Guerino Jr.—was a year older than I. I was nineteen when we got married. We just couldn't wait. I had a two-year college degree when we started our life together. When he died, we'd been married almost twenty-four years. Fredo and I promised each other that we would die together, holding each other in our sleep. We even talked about the date. The first age we picked for dying was one hundred, and then we said, "That's not realistic." So we finally said, "Okay, we'll settle for eighty-two."

We enjoyed life and loved each other desperately. We had a wonderful relationship. But then he died. You just never know. People in the community were surprised, frustrated. It opened a lot of eyes. They never dreamed anything like this would happen to us. We have a very strong Christian family and Christian background. Fredo and I were youth ministers and directors of religious education in addition to our regular jobs. He was an attorney. We did everything together. I worked with him in his law office as a paralegal. Then I continued my degree work and finally became a teacher, a high school teacher, and I absolutely loved that.

Fredo was diagnosed with stomach cancer in November of '96, and he died three months later. He had been healthy and strong that summer. We had done a lot of hard, physical work together in the yard. We had built stone walls and he appeared to be perfectly healthy. There was no indication that anything was wrong. Then he started to get some symptoms. The doctor at first thought it was the flu. It didn't go away. The doctor ran tests for an ulcer, but the tests came back negative. Then the doctor became concerned.

I look back on the time and think how naive and trusting I was. I'll never forget the day I went into the hospital with Fredo for his endoscopy and colonoscopy. They did both tests at the same time. He was pretty much put under, and I was there in the waiting room. I was oblivious. I was happy. I was thinking, "They're going to find what it is and we'll fix it." Then the doctor came out and said, "Diane, I need to talk to you. It's cancer." I had never heard anything so horrible in my life. I just didn't know what to do. I started crying. I was pacing. I said, "What do I do? What do I do?"

They'd been trying to tell Fredo, but he was under so much medication and anesthesia that he wasn't remembering. I was with him in the recovery room and it was late. We were the last appointment of the day. The doctor was due to leave, so I was going to be left there alone with Fredo. I said, "You mean I'm the one who is going to have to tell him?" And he said, "Unfortunately, yes." The doctor had known it was bad as soon as he got in and found the tumor, a gastric adnocarcinoma, a very serious form of cancer. The tumor was very large. The doctor told me that it didn't look good. He didn't hold out a lot of hope even then.

Fredo came from a very large family, nine kids. The doctor said, "Who in the family would people go to if they needed help? That's who you should call now." And I said, "It's Fredo they would go to, but he's in there." Fredo was the rock, the wisdom. When people were in trouble, they would go to him. He was a wise, humble, intelligent man. So I called his brother, Joe, who is my age. He and I have been friends for a very long time. When Joe answered the phone, I couldn't talk. Finally I said, "Joe, it's bad. It's cancer." I decided that I would tell the children myself, that Joe shouldn't take on that responsibility. I would wait for Fredo to wake up, we would discuss it, and then I would go home and tell our three teenagers.

Joe, at that time, was to pick up my daughter for a field hockey banquet at the high school. So he sat through that whole banquet with her, knowing the news but not able to tell her. When I went home, nobody was home yet. But then my son arrived. He was sixteen. He came bouncing into the house and said, "Hi Mom. Where's Dad?" I stood in the doorway and I said, "It's not good, honey. It's cancer." He threw himself on me. He draped himself over me and we stood there and cried. He had questions. I didn't have a lot of answers. Later, both my daughters came home, one after the other, and asked for their father. I told them both the news. All three kids reacted differently. I felt fortunate that I was able to speak to each of them individually. Then I called my parents, who lived an hour away. As soon as they arrived, I packed a few things and went back to the hospital to be with Fredo.

Fredo was in the hospital for about three days for more testing. Then he came home. He seemed the same; it was hard to know that anything serious was wrong. The doctors scheduled surgery to have his stomach removed. They said we'd know after that how serious it really was. They couldn't tell until then. I thought, Okay. Surely this news is going to be good. We had a dose of bad news, but I'm an optimist and a person of faith. I'm thinking, What is God doing? We've lived our lives for God and tried to be good people, and certainly God wouldn't hurt us like this.

Fredo's spirits were pretty optimistic. I was with him every minute that I could be. I took some time off from work. My high school was absolutely wonderful about giving me all the time off that I needed. Fredo had a series of surgeries and chemotherapy, coming home for a week or two, then getting so weak and ill that he had to go back to the hospital for more testing. Sometimes the chemotherapy was so rigorous that he would have to go into the hospital for four or five days for treatment. He had no radiation. Anyway, the surgery news was very bad. It couldn't have been worse. The tumor was very enlarged and had spilled over onto the spleen, so the spleen was involved. We kept thinking, Surely we'll get good news. We'll have good news one of these days. We kept praying. We had thousands of people praying for us. Thousands of letters and cards came in from all over the country. But there were no healing miracles. Every time Fredo went into the hospital, I'd stay with him overnight. He was my best friend in addition to being my husband and a wonderful father. It seemed that his dying process brought us even closer.

In January, the prognosis was getting worse, and they finally told us that they were hoping Fredo would live through spring. I remember sitting with him and finally having discussions about heaven, and that's when we both sort of accepted that this was perhaps what God must want. We were both starting to accept it. Only one time do I remember Fredo crying and saying to me, "Why me? Why am I being taken from you and the kids?" But his faith gave him hope in life beyond this life. He felt that there must be something more for him that God had planned. Just not here. But it hurt him that he had to leave us. And it hurt us, too. Every time he went into the hospital, I would stay with him. I would be as close to him as possible. And if he was at home, I would hold him as much as his physical health allowed. Sometimes he was in pain. I was always trying to rub his back, rub his feet.

Sometimes the medication would make him ache. I wanted to be fully present to him through that process. He accepted that and drew me into the experience with him. He needed it. He wanted it. He knew that I was deeply connected to him in a caring, spiritual sense, which most people didn't even see. But Fredo knew. We gained a profound closeness in sharing an experience like that. It's not an experience anyone would invite, but it drew us very close.

There were times, however, I felt helpless. I remember writing in my journal, "Don't I love him enough that I can make him well?" I would write in my journal every day, and how I was feeling would turn into prayer. I begged God to heal Fredo. I kept thinking about my kids being without their father. I felt that God had given me an overabundance of strength—physical strength, emotional strength, and spiritual strength—that would overflow to Fredo. Fredo knew that, and he loved that about me.

There's no other way for me to explain how I could still do it all—

do a rather adequate job at work, go to the hospital after work, check in with the kids first. I was fortunate enough that the kids were in the high school with me, so that they could see me during the day. At the end of the school day I would spend time with them. Then I would go to the hospital, be with Fredo, sleep in the same bed with him, be as close as I could, take care of whatever needs I could. He loved it when I was there. The next morning, I would get up early, go home, have breakfast with the kids, and then I would be off to work. I did that the entire time, and somehow I had the strength.

Finally in mid-January, our prayers changed from asking God for a healing miracle to asking to accept His will, whatever that might be. The doctors gave us options: no treatment, looking for drugs or treatments around the country, or being treated locally with what they had to offer us, which was a very aggressive regimen. We had developed a really good relationship with our local doctor. We really trusted him. So Fredo chose to be treated locally.

Doug, a close friend of the family, would visit Fredo in the hospital. He came to the house once and brought some medical books. For some reason, at that point, I didn't want to read books about cancer. I was afraid of what I would read. Young Fredo, my son, picked up the books one evening after Dad had gone to bed and he said, "Mom, these are books about people who are dying. Why is he bringing these books into our house?" In reality, Doug knew, the doctors knew. But we continued to just have this little piece of us that didn't want to quite believe what was going happening.

Fredo was at home, in very bad shape. He was weak and having trouble eating. He had a feeding tube. I was taught how to clean it and how to feed him, how to give him the right amount. He had an IV bag hanging by his bed with a timer on it. He couldn't even tolerate that anymore. He couldn't tolerate most things getting into his system. Although he tried to eat, he became more ill. The doctors knew that the cancer had spread. It was everywhere in his abdomen. He was fighting for his life, right from the beginning. The doctors were honest with us. They told us the prognosis was very poor, that he would probably live a year, at best.

Fredo deteriorated quickly. But I look at that now as being a blessing. If he had to die, I can't imagine him suffering any longer than he did. He would have some good days. He would sit in the recliner in the living room. He would walk around a little bit. He never really got outside. He never really got strong enough again to walk up the driveway, even. And that was his goal. He wanted to get outside and enjoy the air. He wanted to see spring. He never had that opportunity. The last time he went into the hospital, he was very weak. I had always been able to handle it before—get him into the car, drive him, park, get him into a wheelchair—and this time I had to call his sister because I couldn't get him up.

That last time we got him into the hospital, they admitted him, actually, to the oncology room where they do chemotherapy. They brought him there, not to the Emergency Room. And at that point, I remember knowing it was serious because Father Nado showed up with the doctor. Fredo was awake. Father Nado was the chaplain at the hospital, a wonderful man who visited Fredo throughout his treatments. The doctor told us it wasn't good. What I don't understand is how he knew. How *do* you know? How do you know you're not going to give him another blood transfusion and we'll have him home? It was at that point that Father Nado gave Fredo his last rites. He was in such poor shape; they didn't know how long he was going to live. It just crushed me. But I had to be strong for Fredo, to give him strength. There were times that we cried together. Often.

He rallied a little bit. Then he sank again. The doctor told us that Fredo might not survive the night. Fredo was conscious but very, very tired. At that point, I made some phone calls and told people that he might not survive the night. *All* of the family arrived at the hospital. They all wanted to have one last moment with Fredo. That was important to Fredo, too. Even to the end, he was concerned about other people's needs, about other people being upset, about other people being sad. Fredo was always helping other people to be strong. People would walk into our home or into his hospital room feeling afraid or weak or sad, not knowing how they were going to deal, and they would walk out feeling stronger. It was amazing.

That night was long and hard. I had the kids come to the hospital first. I took them into a small room and I told them that Daddy was dying. They all fell apart. Even though they knew—they must have known in their hearts—they had been denying it. That night it became real. They all went in with him and they cried with him. He knew what was going on, and he knew that they knew. He apologized and told them how much he loved them. So they spent some time with him, and then they went out, and the rest of the family arrived, our huge family, from both sides. Not only brothers and sisters and spouses but nieces and nephews. It was so important for Fredo to be with them, to be able to say good-bye, to be able to spend a few moments with them.

I have lots of nieces and nephews, too. Fredo would spend a few minutes with each of them, and he had something unique, encouraging, uplifting, and loving to say to each person. A few times toward the end, he said to me, "I can't. The visits are important but I can't do any more." I was the manager of his time that night. I sat through all the visits. I would let him sleep, and then I would rouse him a little bit and ask if he could see so and so. We made it very brief. Everyone was very sensitive, but the hall in the hospital was just filled with people. They would go in and see Fredo, and then they would go out and lose it. There was a lot of sobbing and hugging.

It's amazing how death can draw people closer together. The staff is wonderful on the oncology floor. They're very sensitive to the needs of people who are experiencing cancer treatment. And they're wonderful in the support of families. They're very welcoming of families and anyone who wants to love and support the person through treatment.

Fredo got through that night. He saw every last person. And then, for some reason, the night nurse, the male nurse came in with a blood product for a transfusion. The nurse said, "In the chart it says that if Fredo's reading gets to below a certain point, I'm supposed to order blood products. And that's what I've done." No doctors were there. So the nurse did a blood transfusion on Fredo.

The next morning, Fredo was bright and chipper. We started talking about finances and decisions. He'd say, "Diane, what are you going to do with this?" He was sharp. I had brought the laptop computer for my schoolwork and Fredo said, "Get me the laptop." He had it on the hospital bed. He was sitting up, and we were going through our spreadsheets. He would tell me who to go to for this and that. We went through everything together. I took notes on everything we decided to do. At that point, the reality was unavoidable. Father Nado came in and burst out with a belly laugh. He stood in the doorway and looked at Fredo, bright eyed, with the computer on his lap, and me with a notepad. We were sitting together on the bed, planning as if we were in the law office. The doctors explained later that the blood products had given Fredo a very brief window.

I remember my son struggling. The news was out at school that their dad was dying and then he didn't die. My son came to visit Fredo Sunday. He hugged him and said, "I'm afraid to go back to school. I don't know what the kids will say because—" And his dad said, "Because I was supposed to die and I didn't." And young Fredo said, "Yes."

Fredo said, "Why don't we call Doug? We can watch the films from the last hockey game." My son was playing varsity hockey, and Fredo had missed all the games. Fredo felt bad that he was missing his son's games. So Doug showed up with his fiancée. We never watched the video. Instead, Fredo and Doug talked. Fredo said to him, "Will you watch over young Fredo? He loves you so much. It will make me feel so much better if I know that there's someone at school who will love and support him. I know he has a lot of support at school, but if he can just look in your classroom and make eye contact with you, I'll feel so much better knowing that you're there for him. Will you watch him?" Doug said, "What an honor."

Fredo had a lot of pain swallowing anything, even a sip of water. He had infection inside his system at that point, possibly as a side effect of chemotherapy. He was taking horrible chemicals—poisons. I hated to think of what they were doing to his body. The doctors had said, "Our goal is to have Fredo be well enough to go home and see the spring." They lined up Hospice. They beefed him up. I don't know why. It seemed that the medical attitude changed, perhaps because rotations changed. Certain people had been with us throughout, and all of a sudden there were different faces, different attitudes, different procedures. Doctors even sent in a physical therapist one day who had Fredo do exercises in his bed. The therapist moved his legs up and down, up and down, told him what he should do when he got home. The therapist assumed Fredo was going home.

One morning, at 10:30, after Fredo hadn't been cleaned or been able to shower for a few days, I called the nurse in and said, "Do you think we could give Fredo a sponge bath that would perhaps make him feel better?" So she said, "Why don't we bring him right into the bathroom." He needed help. He was very, very weak. He had his IV pole. We brought him into the bathroom. All of a sudden he said, "I feel like I have to get back to bed. I need to sit down."

So the two of us together got him out the door and he collapsed into a chair. The nurse called the doctors. She went out. More nurses came in. They listened to his heart. They took his blood pressure. They have a blood-pressure monitor. It measured—it's very accurate; you put it on the finger—it measured zero. Zero. They looked at the screen and looked up at me. I knew something was going on, but I wasn't sure what.

One of them went out and brought the doctors in, and we got Fredo into the bed. They checked him over. One of the doctors called me out into the hall and she said, "We're losing him. He may not survive the hour, but we don't know." I said, "Do I have time to contact the kids, to get the kids here?" At that moment one of my very dear friends, who is a nurse at the hospital, showed her face around the corner. She just came to check, to see how we were. I was standing there with the doctor, crying. She said she knew, at that moment. And so I gave her my little phone book and said, "Can you make a few calls?" and then I was back in with Fredo. He was awake. He was able to talk to me. He knew what was going on. He could only talk very quietly, but his mind was still pretty clear.

Uncle Joe got the first call. He went around and gathered up all our kids. He was there it seemed within half an hour. Our kids all have a story of where they were at that moment when they saw Uncle Joe's face in the classroom doorway or wherever they happened to be. And they knew. They came to the hospital, and we all sat around the bed. Then Fredo's brothers and sisters and his dad and my parents and my brothers and sisters all started coming in.

All afternoon, people came in and out. They'd sit there for a while and then leave. Fredo would open his eyes and gaze intently at every individual person in that room. With that gaze, he was saying, "I love you so much." Definitely. And they felt it, I know. Toward the late afternoon, only his dad and my parents were in the room. People were outside in the waiting room or out in the hall. They didn't want to tire Fredo by being present. He was only able to talk to me. He would tell me what he needed, what he wanted to say to someone. But I could tell he was losing energy. He would have to whisper to me. I was standing next to the bed the whole time. And the kids came in and they sat with him. One time, toward the end—we didn't know it was toward the end at that time—one of my daughters came up to me and said, "Mommy, we really want to be here for Daddy, but we're a little bit afraid of what it will be like. Is it okay to be afraid?" She whispered it to me, very quietly. And I told her it was okay. I said, "Listen, honey, I don't know what to expect, either. And Daddy would want you to be comfortable. Whatever you decide is going to be fine. Don't feel guilty. Don't feel afraid. Do what you need to, and it will be just right."

Then Fredo—this is so bizarre—Fredo wanted to take his johnny off. He was pulling at it. He would sit up and lie back. He was restless. He wanted his johnny off. He said he was hot. I took his hospital johnny off. And he had boxers on. The nurse had had to come in earlier to put in a catheter so that he wouldn't have to get up and go to the bathroom. So that was in place. But he kicked the blankets off. Toward the end, he even wanted his boxers off. He was saying he was hot. I tried to convince him that there were people in the room and if he could, it would be better if he could keep his boxers on.

Father Nado came in and saw what Fredo was doing and he said, "Diane, we come into this world naked and we want to leave it naked." Fredo was a very modest man when he was alive and well. He started to moan and complain that the catheter was bothering him. He said, "I have to go to the bathroom." He whispered that to me. I buzzed the nurse. She came in and I told her that he seemed to be having some trouble, some pain. So she said to my parents, Fredo's dad, and the children, "Will you give us just a moment?" So they left.

As soon as the door closed, he started to breathe very heavily, and I said, "He hasn't done this before. He hasn't done this today." The nurse looked at me and she said, "He's leaving us."

Fredo was breathing very, very erratically. It was like he'd waited to be alone with me. So I went to Fredo—I mean, I went right to his face. I'll never forget it. I was whispering in his ear as he was going. I was saying, "Fredo, I love you so much, and I'll miss you so much. But I know you have to go. You'll finally get to see the Lord's face. What a gift." I kept saying those things to him. I knew he loved the Lord so much, and I knew where he was going that he would be okay and we would always love him. I told him all those things. I kept saying those things to him over and over and over again. I was crying, but I was able to talk. I was holding his face with one hand, holding his shoulder. I was so close to him, as close as I could be. How can you plan a moment like that? You can't. You can't plan a moment like that. It was just instinct. It was natural.

I was so close to Fredo that I wanted to be right there with him as he crossed over—whatever crossing over is. I was right there with him during his leaving. That, to me, is one of the greatest gifts I ever had. He could have gone in the night while I was sleeping in the cot next to him. He could have gone at any time. Fredo died at 4:30 in the afternoon. The doctor had to come in and pronounce the time. Then the kids and Fredo's dad came in. The kids and I merged into one being. We were hugging each other, holding each other, and sobbing. Then Grandpa Guerino came up and put his arms around all of us and we knew it was finished. People started leaving. Some people came in to see him for one last time. Others couldn't. Then people started going home, and it was just the five of us. The kids and I sat around his bed with him. He looked so peaceful. The kids weren't afraid of him at that point. It was very peaceful. We were sitting there, and we weren't crying. Father Nado came in and said, "I think it's time." He had to help us identify that it was time to leave, that it was okay to leave. Do you know? It's like we just wanted to sit there with him. I don't know how long we would have done that.

The kids helped me pack up all my stuff—I had had books there and clothes. I had moved in. They all hugged me and cried and said, "It will be so nice to have you home again, Mommy. We've missed you. We've missed you so much."

I'll never forget that last walk down the corridor of that hospital, down the hall of the oncology ward, with the four of us clinging, hugging, our arms around each other's necks and arms and backs, all four of us walking together, away from that place. I'll never forget that. It was as if, Okay, now it's us. A brother-in-law was waiting for us right at the entry, and he took us home. That was a tough night. It had been very hard to leave that room. Very hard.

At the funeral, the church was packed to the brim. The hardest part was when the casket was rolled down the aisle and we came out of our pew and followed. There was something about that moment that really hit me, and made me realize, This is it. He's not coming back. I think maybe I was in shock before then. But that moment really affected me. It wasn't at the cemetery. It wasn't at the wake. It was at that moment, when we followed his casket out of the church. I walked out with Fredo's dad, my arm in his arm, and the three kids behind us all crying. I remember turning around. I kept turning around and turning around and turning around, looking at them, touching them.

I can tell you the moment—I know the exact moment when Fredo's spirit departed. I wrote about it in my journal. It was on what would have been our twenty-fifth wedding anniversary last June. I went to the grave site and put a dozen long-stemmed roses on his grave. I have to say that I still felt desperately connected to him. I felt a spiritual awareness or presence that I could still be desperately in love with. I don't know that many people would understand what I mean by that. But I still felt that it was all right to love him as I had for the better part of my life. I assumed that I would live alone for the rest of my life with wonderful memories, pouring my love into my children and eventually becoming a grandmother.

And I started to say to God, "I can love Fredo forever. If it's what you want for my life, then give me the strength and the courage." I was involved in a lot of community activities. I was friends with some wonderful men. But they were never anything other than acquaintances or friends. I envisioned myself being like that forever, just feeling complete with wonderful friends and my kids. And I wrote, "Our twenty-fifth wedding anniversary. Shattered dreams, a broken heart, so lonely for Fredo. No will ever take his place. We had the very best marriage. When a woman spends the better part of her life loving one man, being completely committed to him—when he is suddenly gone, never to return—she is left with cherished memories and broken dreams. She is left with a confused sense of self and purpose. All the love, all the energy, all the laughter, all the passion that was expended on loving her husband—where does all of that go? It leaves a hole in her soul, a gaping, open wound that refuses to heal. Today I will put a dozen red roses at your grave. I will remember the beautiful life that we shared, and I will continue to miss your face, your voice, your laugh, your touch. Fredo Guerino, I still love you so much."

That's what I was feeling. That's where my heart was at that time. And when I went to his grave, I sensed that he knew it. But for the very first time, when I walked away from his grave, something different happened in my heart, mind, and soul. It wasn't obvious. It was just this small thing, a question. I remember getting in the car, driving home, and thinking, Is this a healthy place for me to be? Am I stuck?

I never thought I would have asked that question. Later, I went to see our friend, Doug. I said to him, "How long can a woman desperately love a man who has died?" I don't remember what Doug said back to me. What was more important was that I was asking the question.

Ira Byock, M.D.

I originally learned about Dr. Ira Byock through reading his book, *Dying Well.*
The book made a significant contribution to the literature of the field and to
my own life. The personal warmth, compassion, and wisdom in his book
inspired me to seek him out and to include his thoughts about death in this
book. When I located him, Ira was working as director of the Palliative Care
Service in Missoula, Montana. He has since moved to the East Coast, where he
is now director of Palliative Medicine at Dartmouth-Hitchcock Medical Center
in Lebanon, New Hampshire, and a professor at Dartmouth Medical School.
His latest book is *The Four Things That Matter Most.*

I don't really know a hoot about death. Never been there. As I
understand it, at least with my present level of human consciousness—and I would submit the majority of human consciousness—it
is genuinely unknowable. We can make some inferences from what
we do know, but frankly, death is unknowable. I don't understand it
at all. I have some thoughts about it, though, but they're in the
realm of the metaphysical. I rarely talk about death, frankly, because
I want to preserve my credibility as a physician, as a researcher.

I don't really feel that I am an expert about dying, but I am a very
deliberate, serious student. The more mysterious questions I have to
label as beliefs, as interpretations, but not as something that comes
from direct experience. And yet it does, but not in the sense that I
can assert it to others.

The fact of the matter is that the moment of death and the events around death strip away the cloak of illusion that surrounds our experience of life. We cloak ourselves with illusion that we are discrete, that we are individuals, independent of others, living an independent life as an individual. But in fact, nothing could be further from the truth. And here's where the philosophical, the metaphysical, converges on the concrete.

It may be rooted in our biology as mammals to believe ourselves to be discrete. It may be an adaptive illusion that is necessary for the survival of the species or that at least has been necessary for the survival of the species. We have to know who is hungry, to eat. We have to know who fears death, to avoid dying, or we won't live to pass on our genes. Right? In fact, we are not discrete. We are intimately connected.

It is not merely death and the moment of death that is sacred. If we can see the world in real clarity, it is all of life and existence itself that is sacred. What death does is this: at the moment of death, we are with someone who is there and is part of our universe and then who is not there. In seeing them approach that transition with—at least from our external observations—this sense of utter clarity and acceptance at that last moment, this sense of transcendence, it parts the curtains and allows us to see things clearly. And what we see is that life is not what it appears to be on a busy Wednesday afternoon. It is not what it appears.

We contemporaries, we moderns are particularly deluded in this notion that reality is what we can see and touch. We think that our lives as individuals are long and real and that that's what reality is. And we say everything else is religion or philosophy or metaphysics. Just think about it. Let's think about what we know.

For one thing, here we are, all six billion of us, clinging to the surface of what is genuinely a rock hurtling through deep space. The circumference of our planet is what? Twenty-seven thousand miles at its widest point. My Saab has traveled six times that number of miles. This earth is a small place. And we're hurtling through a galaxy and a universe that is unimaginably large. We are held to the surface of our planet by something we are told to call gravity, whatever the hell that is—an attraction of bodies for each other. We are separated from the cold void of space by the thinnest of gaseous cushions. I would submit that we live in an illusion. We live in an illusion of our separateness, of our durability as individuals, when in fact we are naked to the universe and to the infinite, in so many ways.

In truth, we are intimately connected to each other. If you look at what we know now about ecology and also about social biology, about quantum mechanics in physics, about any stream of scientific investigation that in any way involves human life, and you take it far enough, you come to a point at which we are genuinely interconnected in an inextricable way. The very meaning of being human, in fact, from a social-psychology perspective, entails a sense of connectedness. That often becomes very clear around terminal illness.

People say to me, "My stepfather is ill in Ohio, and I don't know whether to visit or not. Personally, I don't know if I can stand it. And I don't know if I would be intruding or not." Usually I ask them, "Well, what's your relationship? How close have you been?" And the person says, "Well, actually we grew pretty close. Never superclose, but we were friends." Then the person might tell me a story of a trip they'd taken together or things that they had shared or a car they had fixed together or something.

What I try to reflect back to them is that this situation is not something you can avoid by denying it's happening and thereby keeping yourself distant. When to go back to visit or how intimately to be involved in the dying person's process is something friends and relatives have to feel out. But frankly, if you know this person, if you have affection for this person and you know of their illness and impending death, you already own this pain. You can't avoid it. You can only choose how directly to deal with it.

Whatever you know, the dying person also knows on some level. So my usual suggestion is to err on the side of checking in, of maybe even of showing up. And if it's uncomfortable, well, then at that point it will become clearer to you. But knowing what I know about our culture, I would say "Go. Check in. Make the call. State the obvious." What I mean by that is: name your own feelings. People can simply say to a dying person, "It was hard for me to even hear about it. It was painful to me to hear that you were ill," or "I'm really worried. I wanted to be here. It was important for me," or, "It scares me to think that you might die."

I think it's important to discuss death in terms of "I" statements—naming your own needs, worries, concerns, and feelings. We're on a lot safer ground when we make sure that our motives are really coming out of genuine love for the other person, that we're not in some way feeding our needs by needing the ill person to say something to us or having expectations that the ill person should approach the end of life in some specific way. I worry when people go with an agenda to help people accept what's happening. The sick person has to accept death or not accept it. You should go and express your concern. You can simply be present to help, to take out the garbage, to cook up meals. Just show up and say the obvious, which is, "I love you and I'm worried about you and I needed to see you because I love you." That's all okay.

You can make it clear to people who are dying that you're willing and able to listen to whatever they have to say. You can make it safe for them to speak about their fears. To do that, you have to get pretty clear inside that you would be available for that. It takes some intentionality. It takes some preparation. What am I going to say if Ed says to me, "I just want to die"? Or what will I say if he says to me, "I really wish somebody would shoot me." Or he says to me, "I just feel like I'm a burden. I'm just sitting here waiting to die." What are you going to say back? You don't need to have answers, by the way. But you need to be able to be present without saying, "Oh, don't talk like that," without running away. It's a perfectly fine answer to say "I don't know," or "Gee, this stuff is hard." That's a good answer. State the obvious.

It is a privilege to be present for death. It's a privilege to be present beforehand as well. The privilege comes partly from the fact that death strips away the illusions and makes clearer how precious every fleeting moment of life is. It doesn't make life more precious, but it provides a background against which we can see the preciousness of life. We can come out of the illusion that life is long and that we can confidently expect tomorrow and next year. That's all important to living fully and being adaptable, but it's also an illusion.

Do I have any insight as a physician? No I don't, as a physician. I can explain a fair amount about the mechanisms of cellular death, but why all the systems that were working stopped working is a mystery. Frankly, it's not as much of a mystery as why those systems were working in the first place—honestly. And again, that's the more miraculous thing. Why do all these structures exist at all and why is *life* the synthetic result of putting this human structure together? Why? What is *that*? What *is* that? Life is really the truly miraculous thing. Whether it is articulated in that sense or not, that is what death reveals: the improbability and miracle that life itself is.

Having said that, I don't know where the electrons go, where the energy, the spirit, the soul go, when somebody dies. Whether it's spirit or soul or *chi*, I don't know. I have a sense—not from my doctorness or anything scientific—but a strong intuitive sense as a very serious student of the workings of the universe, to the extent that my intellectual capabilities and limitations allow, that the density of consciousness that life and certainly mammalian life or human life represents is not completely dissolved, does not vanish, at death.

It seems to me consistent with what I know about the rest of this universe that in some way this concentration of consciousness is reorganized, transformed, and exists in some other fashion. It seems very unlikely to me that it simply vanishes as if it never was. Beyond that, I can explain some of the theories I've read as to what happens, but I *do not know*. I do not know. I do think that we're connected and that we're connected on a lot of levels. A lot of those levels are ones that we simply do not understand in the current form of our human existence.

I cannot explain so many of the stories I have heard where people at a great distance have a profound feeling, an unmistakable awareness of another person and of their dying, often hours before—sometimes days before—they find out that indeed at that time the person was dying or had died. But I've heard dozens of these stories. I can't explain them, but I do believe them. In fact it would be silly to not believe them simply because we cannot explain them. They're too consistent. And they come from people who have no reason in any way to mislead or to make up these things. These stories are not fantasy. I think that they are one of the little pieces of empirical evidence that life is more than it appears on the surface, that this life—our current physical existence—is not all there is. Beyond that, I don't know.

People come back to people in dreams, too. After someone has died that person comes to other people in profound dreams. I don't know what to make of that either. In the dreams, I've been told, there are some concrete factual collaborations or extreme associations; you have to believe or not believe them. But there certainly is a strong pattern to those sorts of things.

I knew of a young man who died, who actually collapsed at a bowling alley. He was in his late twenties or early thirties, a strong, strapping, healthy guy. He just dropped dead at the bowling alley. They resuscitated him and brought him to the hospital. He never regained consciousness. He ended up with only his brain stem functioning—a variant of a persistent, vegetative state. His eyes were open, but nothing above the brain stem was really working. On the basis of a physical exam, of the EEG, there was no cortical activity. This is really remarkable. He didn't even have heart disease. They really didn't have a reason for him to die. They did coronary angiography on this guy, but there was nothing there. It happened in another town, but he was transferred to Missoula, where he and his wife lived. He had been in the other town for a pool tournament that was being held at a bowling alley.

I got involved. I saw the patient and family when he was in a nursing home. Three or four weeks after this event, he was still alive, and his wife had decided that she would like to pull the feeding tube. She and her doctor had worked through that. She had power of attorney and his family, his mom and dad, had come out from somewhere in Minnesota to be with him. The feeding tube was pulled and he was referred to Hospice.

I was working with Hospice at the time, and that was how I got to see him. His doctor had gone out of town, and I was asked to check in on him from time to time. I went over there. The feeding tube had been out for something like four or five days, and there were the inevitable questions, such as, "How long will he live?"

I checked him over. His heart rate was normal and his urine output was good, his skin was moist. I'd written in the chart that I thought that given his general state of health and his level of hydration and all before this happened that it was likely that he was going to live quite possibly another week. His family wasn't there. They'd stepped out of the room when I saw him. I wrote them a note.

When I went back to check on him, his mom and dad were there. They had come back in, and his mom was at the head of his bed. She was mopping his brow. He was sort of almost a little sweaty. His dad was standing there by the side of the bed. I met them and said who I was and why I was there.

I said, "Is there anything I can do for you?" I told them what was happening. I told them that I didn't think their son was suffering. I told them that I was really, really sorry this happened but that as far as I could determine, there was no distress. I said, "Can you think of anything else that I or the Hospice team can be doing?" Their first answer was no, that things were going as well as could be expected. "It's really hard, but no, thank you, Doctor." And then his father said, "There is one thing you could do." And he looked at me and he said, "No. Well, there is one thing you could do, but I know you won't."

We looked at each other. I thought I knew what he meant, but I intended only to be present—as the expression goes—"Stay close and do nothing." So I held his gaze and said, "I can only guess. What do you mean? What do you think I might do?" And he said, "Well, you could get this over with." And I said, "If you mean to give your son something to end his life now, you're right, it's something I can't do."

I said, "You know, I've reviewed his chart carefully, and I'll tell you, in reviewing it, my heart aches. I have no idea why your son had his heart attack, why his heart stopped. And frankly, since that happened, I have no idea why he's still alive. I don't have an answer for that. I know that in reviewing this case before coming here and in the conversations we've had in Hospice, I know that you've had the opportunity to come out and at least be with him and didn't have to get the call that he was dead. Maybe there was some value in at least his living that long. And I know, now that you've come, that you've had a chance to be with his wife, to be here, and to support her."

And the father said, "Yes. We've had a chance to meet a lot of his friends and through his friends to get a sense of who he was and to know our son in a way we frankly hadn't in the past. I have to tell you, Doc, it has been a couple of remarkable weeks for us. It makes us sad, but it has been remarkable."

And I said, "So I don't know why he's still alive. I just assessed him, and I think he's going to be alive for several days to come. Because he's so strong and he's actually such a healthy guy, it seems paradoxical to say, but he's been so healthy that I don't think he's going to die suddenly here. Maybe he's been hanging around." And I said this with a facial expression that let them know that I was just sort of saying this in a metaphorical or a metaphysical sense. "Maybe he's hanging around so that you have the opportunity to kind of adjust to this a little bit. But I don't know." And the father got tearful, and his wife got tearful.

The father said, "You know, this has been extraordinary. I don't know why, but this has been a very important time for us. Thanks, Doc. Thanks a lot for taking such good care of him and of us." I told them that I would be available and would check back and that we certainly weren't going to let their son suffer, that I was going to treat him as my own brother. Then I left and drove back to my office, ten minutes away. I got back to the office, and I walked in the door. The phone was ringing. He had just died.

Now, go figure. I don't have any data here except for the story. We humans are meaning makers. We can't help it. We search for meaning. It's biological. But to me, I have to wonder whether that young man was not in some sense hovering, as so often people do who come back from near-death experiences. I have to wonder whether he wasn't in the room, listening, watching, and deciding at that point that he could go.

I certainly have seen a large handful of people die within a few minutes of having been given permission to die. I've *certainly* seen people change. Many times you see people change from distress to a more peaceful physiology, pulse and respiration, less muscle tightness, when they are given permission to die. "It's okay, Dad. Everything's all right. We're all here. We've taken care of things. We love you. We'll miss you, but you can go." That's *so* common that to think that that's not real would be folly. I can't explain the phenomenon, but I do think it's real. I also believe that people can delay their death and that they can will themselves to die more quickly. There's no question about that. In one sense, in the course of a chronic illness and maybe more generally, people almost have to decide when it's their time to die.

If we were to see the world utterly and clearly, we would recognize the privilege of being with another person for *every* moment. We would see that in a sense the time we call dying is not special. Death is a moment that we share with one another that is miraculous—because every moment is. Life is indeed sacred and miraculous and precious. Now I know, saying that, that I'm sounding like a religious monk or a mystic or the Dalai Lama. But in fact I really think that that is what death reveals to us.

The word *sacred* comes up a lot. I think of it when I walk into the home of someone who is dying. There is a sacredness there that is every bit as powerful and palpable as the feelings that I get in the Notre Dame cathedral in Paris or listening to the Dalai Lama, or Beethoven's Ninth or Bach's cello suites or fugues or reading from the great books of the world, the *Bhagavad Gita* or the *Bible* or the *Koran*. There is a sense at that bedside, in that house, that there's an awareness that something precious is happening, that this is a very special time. Several times, there is an odd mixture of solemnity and celebration that I feel often in these situations. There is a remarkable celebration of life—of one particular life but also of life in relationship with one another. That celebration is evident despite everyone's obvious acknowledgment of the sadness of the situation.

Look at what the Buddhists do. The more observant Buddhists are, the more they talk about the preciousness of every moment of life. They sit with the body nine days, but they begin with real attention to that transition. They meditate on the body, meditate on the physical body as it begins to decay, meditate on the transience of life—which is, I would submit, doing exercises in piercing our illusions of mortality. The reverence for life that arises from that approach is profound.

MARJORIE RYERSON, an award-winning journalist and professor of journalism at Castleton State College, is also a photographer and a poet. She is the author of the photography book *Water Music* (University of Michigan Press, 2003) and executive director of the nonprofit organization Water Music, Inc. (www.water-music.org). She also teaches poetry for Middlebury College's New England Young Writers' Conference at Bread Loaf and runs workshops in writing about grief and loss. Ryerson's photographs and news and feature stories have appeared in numerous magazines, books, and newspapers across the Northeast for the past twenty-five years. She was honored as the Vermont State Colleges' Faculty Fellow for 2000–2001 and won the 2004 Paul Keough Award for leadership in the water environment. She lives in Vermont.